The Bi-Personal Field

In *The Bi-Personal Field: Experiences in Child Analysis* Antonino Ferro sets out his new conceptual system for analysis, considering not only the inner world of the patient but the continued interaction of that world with the inner world of the analyst.

The book takes a fresh look at the main aspects of theory and technique in psychoanalysis in the light of Kleinian developments, in particular reflecting the drastic changes due to the thinking of Bion. Illustrated with numerous detailed clinical examples, the author claims that the basic focus of the analytic relationship is the conscious and unconscious interpersonal/intersubjective processes going on between the analyst and patient.

Antonino Ferro is Supervisor at the 'Dosso Verde' Child Psychotherapy Centre, Pavia University. He is also Visiting Professor of Child Psychotherapy and Psychoanalysis at Milan University, and a psychoanalyst in private practice.

THE NEW LIBRARY OF PSYCHOANALYSIS

The New Library of Psychoanalysis was launched in 1987 in association with the Institute of Psycho-Analysis, London. Its purpose is to facilitate a greater and more widespread appreciation of what psychoanalysis is really about and to provide a forum for increasing mutual understanding between psychoanalysts and those working in other disciplines such as history, linguistics, literature, medicine, philosophy, psychology and the social sciences. It is intended that the titles selected for publication in the series should deepen and develop psychoanalytic thinking and technique, contribute to psychoanalysis from outside, or contribute to other disciplines from a psychoanalytical perspective.

The Institute, together with the British Psycho-Analytical Society, runs a low-fee psychoanalytic clinic, organizes lectures and scientific events concerned with psychoanalysis, publishes the *International Journal of Psycho-Analysis* (which now incorporates the *International Review of Psycho-Analysis*), and runs the only training course in the UK in psychoanalysis leading to membership of the International Psychoanalytical Association – the body which preserves internationally agreed standards of training, of professional entry, and of professional ethics and practice for psychoanalysis as initiated and developed by Sigmund Freud. Distinguished members of the Institute have included Michael Balint, Wilfred Bion, Ronald Fairbairn, Anna Freud, Ernest Jones, Melanie Klein, John Rickman and Donald Winnicott.

Volumes 1–11 in the series have been prepared under the general editorship of David Tuckett, with Ronald Britton and Eglé Laufer as associate editors. Subsequent volumes are under the general editorship of Elizabeth Bott Spillius, with, from Volume 17, Donald Campbell, Michael Parsons, Rosine Jozef Perelberg and David Taylor as associate editors.

ALSO IN THIS SERIES

NEW LIBRARY OF PSYCHOANALYSIS
——38——

General editor: Elizabeth Bott Spillius

The Bi-Personal Field

EXPERIENCES IN CHILD ANALYSIS

ANTONINO FERRO

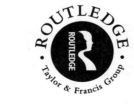

London and New York

First published 1999
by Routledge
11 New Fetter Lane, London EC4P 4EE

Simultaneously published in the USA and Canada
by Routledge
29 West 35th Street, New York, NY 10001

Routledge is an imprint of the Taylor & Francis Group

Originally published in 1992 as *La tecnica nella psicoanalisi infantile: Il
bambino e l'analista: dalla relazione al campo emotivo*

Typeset in Bembo by J&L Composition Ltd, Filey, North Yorkshire
Printed and bound in Great Britain by
MPG Book Ltd, Bodmin

British Library Cataloguing in Publication Data
A catalogue record for this book is available from the British Library

Library of Congress Cataloging in Publication Data
Ferro, Antonino, 1947–
[Tecnica nella psicoanalisi infantile. English]
The bi-personal field: experiences in child analysis / Antonino Ferro.
p. cm. – (New library of psychoanalysis: 38)
Includes bibliographical references and index.
1. Child analysis. 2. Child psychiatry. 3. Psychotherapist and patient.
4. Psychoanalysis–Philosophy. I. Title. II. Series.
[DNLM: 1. Psychoanalysis – in infancy & childhood.
2. Psychoanalysis – methods. 3. Psychoanalytic Theory.   W1 NE455F
v.36   1999 / WS 350.5 F395t 1999]
RJ504.2.F4713   1999
618.92'8917—dc21
DNLM/DLC
for Library of Congress 98–52402
CIP

ISBN 0–415–21179–4 (hbk)
ISBN 0–415–21180–8 (pbk)

Contents

Acknowledgements

I would like to give particular thanks to Elizabeth Bott Spillius and John Coggan without whose very careful and caring help this book would not have seen the light of day.

Introduction

ELIZABETH BOTT SPILLIUS

Dr Antonino Ferro, a distinguished Italian analyst, studied medicine and psychiatry at Palermo and psychoanalysis at the Milan Institute of Psychoanalysis. He is a training analyst of the Italian Psychoanalytical Society, Visiting Professor of Psychiatric Semiotics in Pavia University and of Child Psychotherapy at Milan University. He has worked together closely with a group of Milan colleagues, particularly Giuseppe Di Chiara, Luciana Nissim Momigliano, Eugenio Gaburri, and Dina Vallino Macciò, and also with Michele Bezoari in Pavia.

As the reader will soon discover from reading the abundant clinical presentations of this book, Dr Ferro has the gift of clinical imagination, a marked capacity to sense the thoughts and feelings of the other person and to feel how they relate to his own. He has worked particularly with children – those forthright critics of adult pretensions – but, like Klein and Bion before him, he sees no difference in the basic approach and technique of psychoanalysis with children and with adults. Psychoanalysis is one.

Ferro attempts to develop a new conceptual system to express and contain his clinical approach. In the first chapter of this book he describes, as he sees them, the basic tenets of the conceptual schemes of Freud, Klein, and, using the ideas of Bion and Willy and Madeleine Baranger, *the bi-personal field*, the conceptualization that he and some of his colleagues have developed.

In Freud's system, according to Ferro, the basic focus is on the conscious and unconscious effects of the patient's history and external relations; in Klein's system, it is on the patient's intrapsychic world of unconscious phantasy; in his own, it is on the conscious and unconscious interpersonal/ intersubjective processes going on between analyst and patient. It will be clear even from this skeletal description that Ferro's approach has certain features in common with some of the exponents of self-psychology, relational analysis, social constructivism and intersubjectivism in the USA. He differs from them in important respects, however. I believe that the various schools of thought mentioned above have been influenced mainly by Kohut and the ideas of self-psychology as well as by Harry Stack Sullivan, whereas Ferro's formulations derive mainly from Bion and the Barangers. A further difference is that Ferro presents far more clinical material than most American psychoanalysts, so that it is easy to compare what he and his patients say and do with his conceptual formulations.

Ferro takes it more or less for granted that the ordinary psychoanalytic/ psychotherapeutic reader will understand the ideas of Bion, so that I think at least a brief description of some of Bion's views may be useful here for those readers who come from a different psychoanalytic tradition.

Ostensibly Bion's work is concerned with 'thinking' and indeed he developed many of his ideas in the psychoanalytic study of thought disorders in schizophrenic patients. But in Bion's approach 'thinking' includes 'feeling', so that it is far from being an exercise in logic alone. Bion's work is built on that of Klein, especially on her notion of *projective identification* (Klein 1946), which Bion greatly extended, and on the ideas of the *paranoid-schizoid* and *depressive positions* (Klein 1935, 1940, 1946). Ferro's view is that Bion's development of Klein's work is so extensive that his is a completely new, 'non-Kleinian' approach. My own view and that of many of my colleagues (and of Bléandonu 1994) is that Bion's work is a very productive development of Klein's thought, and that most Kleinian analysts today have adopted many of Bion's views. But this question of whether Bion is 'Kleinian' or not is a minor issue. It is his ideas that matter.

Klein's idea of projective identification is that an individual may split off certain aspects of himself, his thoughts and feelings and project them in phantasy into another person – in the analytic situation, into the analyst. He then perceives the analyst as the repudiated aspects of himself. The projected aspects may be 'good' or 'bad', though the projection of bad aspects has been much more discussed than the projection of good aspects. Klein did not believe that the analyst should be emotionally influenced by these projections, which fundamentally were in her view only a phantasy of the patient; if the analyst was influenced it was a sign that he needed more analysis. In a similar way she did not think that the analyst's countertransference could be a useful source of information about the patient. On the contrary, as she dryly put it on one occasion, it was a useful source of information about the analyst (Klein 1958).

Bion took the concept of projective identification much further than Klein and changed its clinical significance, for he thought that it was a basic mode of communication between mother and infant and later, between any two people, including analyst and patient, and within and between groups (Bion 1959, 1961, 1962a, b). He distinguished between 'normal' and 'pathological' projective identification and his work on both types set the stage for regarding the analytic dyad as a potential field of mutual projection. All current Kleinian analysts have followed Bion's lead in using his idea that an important part of the analytic process is that the analyst will be emotionally influenced by the patient's projections. Optimally, the analyst will be able to use his responses to these projections to understand his patient better. The hazard is that the analyst will be threatened by the patient's projection and will unconsciously block it, or, if he allows it into his mind, he will be overwhelmed by it so that he cannot think, or so that he will withdraw emotionally or resort to some form of unproductive acting out in the session.

Bion uses this model of response to projection to present a theory of the development of thinking based on what he calls the '*container/contained*' ($♀/♂$), in which the 'container' represents the receptive mind capable of what he calls '*reverie*' such that it is able to 'contain' the contents that are projected into it. In Bion's view the aim of the receptive mind is, through reverie, to transform the 'contained' into a form that the original projector may be able to take back into his own mind.

Bion distinguishes between what he calls '*beta*' elements and '*alpha*' elements. Beta elements are indigestible experiences or raw sensations that cannot be thought about or used for thinking; they are, as Bion puts it, fit only for evacuation. Alpha elements are beta elements that have been modified by 'alpha function' (containment and transformation) so that they can be used as the raw materials for dream and for thought. Ferro speaks of '*alphabetization*', meaning the process by which beta elements are converted into alpha elements. He also makes it clear, following Meltzer (1978: Part 3, Chapter 5), that optimally alphabetization goes on as an unconscious process all the time in everyone's mind; it is the unconscious daytime form of dreaming.

Two other ideas are crucial in Bion's thought and are currently much used by his Kleinian colleagues in Britain and elsewhere: the idea of fluctuation between the paranoid-schizoid and the depressive position ($PS \longleftrightarrow D$) and the idea of K and $-K$. Klein originally thought of the paranoid-schizoid position as a stage of development in early infancy in which good and bad experiences were kept separate, an important development for the establishment of differentiation of experiences and hence, later, for the experience of integrating them. The depressive position she thought occurred at a slightly later period in infancy and she believed that it involved the integration of the good and the bad object which had formerly been felt to be completely separate, so that the infant now came to realize that the mother he hated and the mother he loved were one and the same person. Among Klein's current colleagues the recognition of the object's and one's own separateness has come to be regarded as an equally important aspect of the depressive position. Further, Klein linked the depressive position with early stages of the Oedipus complex, and this aspect too has been increasingly emphasized by many current Kleinian analysts, especially Ronald Britton (1989).

Klein thought of the paranoid-schizoid and depressive positions as normal phases of development, but called them '*positions*' to emphasize that some movement between them continued throughout life. Bion greatly increased use of the idea of fluctuation between the paranoid-schizoid and depressive positions, including the idea that there are positive elements in the paranoid-schizoid position and negative elements in the depressive position. Hence the aim of psychoanalytic therapy is no longer phrased by Bion, nor, in spite of Ferro's statement to the contrary, by most Kleinian analysts at the present time, as the 'achievement' of the depressive position. Ferro describes his view of the aim of psychoanalytic therapy, and I think Bion and current Kleinian analysts would agree, as making it possible for the patient to 'think' better, meaning that his capacity for containment would be enlarged.

In addition to the usual drives of love and hate, Bion assumes that there is a drive to *know*, which he designates as 'K', and, equally important, a drive *to destroy knowing*, which he designates as '$-K$'. A person in the grip of $-K$ dismantles knowing, attacks it, or converts it into possession of knowledge rather than the process of coming to know new experiences. In describing processes of child–mother or patient–analyst interaction, Bion assumes that the outcome depends not only on the mother's or analyst's capacity for reverie and K but also on the balance of K and $-K$ in the child or patient.

In his later work (post-1970) Bion focuses more and more on the psychoanalytic process itself and on the mind of the analyst in it. He begins to emphasize not only the analyst's capacity for reverie but also, as Ferro frequently mentions, the role of the patient as the analyst's 'best colleague' (Bion 1980) in pointing out, directly or symbolically, the analyst's weaknesses and strengths. Ferro considers it to be a leitmotif of all Bion's work that he conceived of the analyst's mind, its function and dysfunction, to be powerfully present in the psychoanalytic process. Projective identifications, Ferro goes on to say, are not the prerogative of the patient. 'They are also a perfectly normal way for human minds to communicate. It follows, then, that they are reciprocal and intersecting' (Chapter 1).

Ferro notes, too, that Bion is less interested in content than in what, following Freud, he calls the 'mental apparatus', that is, the mind itself. Bion views the aim of analysis as the growth of the mind and its capacity to contain and develop thoughts. Ferro, like Meltzer, regards the analytic couple as a group of two and regards the aim of the analytic process as the expansion and development of the minds of both members. Further, Bion lays increasing stress on the importance of '*unsaturated*' thoughts and interpretations that allow the patient to develop a thought further. Ferro and

Bezoari (1989) call such interpretations 'weak' (in the philosophical sense), contrasting them with 'strong' (or closed) interpretations which allow the patient little room to make his own contribution and which locate all cleverness and insight in the analyst.

Ferro and his colleagues have made considerable use not only of the ideas of Bion but also those of Willy and Madeleine Baranger, South American analysts of French origin who were trained in psychoanalysis in Buenos Aires and then worked in Argentina and Uruguay. Their work does much to link the approaches of Kleinian analysis and Gestalt psychology. Following the ideas of Kurt Lewin (1935, 1952), they regard the clinical situation of psychoanalysis as a '*bi-personal field*' shaped by both participants and, specifically, shaped by the projections of both participants. This formulation is close to the 'analytic third' idea of Ogden (1994), though to my way of thinking it is less mystical, less difficult to analyse into its component parts. The Barangers assume that most of the time an analysis goes along more or less satisfactorily with the analyst being able to use his capacity for reverie to modify the patient's projections. Every now and again, however, the analysis gets stuck, usually through a shared phantasy or dovetailing phantasies taking possession of analyst and patient in such a fashion that they develop a state of unconscious collusion with each other. Such stuck states the Barangers refer to as '*bastions*', and they suggest that the analyst then needs to take what they call a '*second glance*' to analyse his own involvement in the bastion and through doing so to release the imprisoned analytic process.

Ferro points out, however, that the Barangers differ from Bion (and from Ferro himself at what he regards as his best) in that they make '*strong*' or '*saturated*' interpretations in which, like Freud and Klein in Ferro's view, they regard it as proper analytic technique to decode meanings, although in this case it is the meaning of the shared phantasy that needs interpretation rather than the unconscious phantasy of the patient (Klein) or the historical/ internal/external conflicts of the patient (Freud).

For Ferro and his colleagues the understanding of what is going on in the bi-personal field remains, as Ferro and Bezoari put it 'a *fil rouge* in the analyst's mind – a real Ariadne's threat that helps him not to lose his way – but also a condition in which meaning is allowed to develop freely during the session' (Bezoari and Ferro 1992: 57). In this stress Ferro has much in common with the certain American schools of thought, as I have noted above. He shares with them a dislike of saturated or authoritative interpretations which decode meanings and reveal truths about the patient, especially interpretations that 'blame' the patient and elevate the analyst, an attitude that Ferro implies is sometimes found in Freudian and Kleinian analysts – though he also makes clear that he himself makes 'decoding' interpretations at times. But Ferro's approach to the analytic process lays considerable stress, more stress than that described by most American relational analysts and intersubjectivists, on asymmetry in the roles of patient and analyst. In spite of mutual subjective involvement the analyst, in Ferro's view, has a special responsibility in the dyad, which makes his role markedly different from that of the patient. It is the analyst's responsibility to protect the patient from his (the analyst's) projections and to develop and strengthen the patient's capacity to think. Basically, though Ferro does not put it this way, the patient is there to be understood, the analyst is there to understand, though much inevitable mutuality must go on in the process of reaching understanding.

Ferro has developed an idiosyncratic and to me somewhat impenetrable vocabulary for describing certain features of the bi-personal field: *'characters'*, *'functional aggregates'*, *'affective holograms'*. *'Character'*, as I understand it, may be a particular personification in the patient's material, but it may also be a quality in the analyst–patient relationship. In response to my query about it Ferro described the idea of 'character' as follows:

> If a patient keeps talking about his/her 'cat', one model suggests we interpret it as a real external cat, with all the feelings and emotions this cat may have, including memories of kittenhood, family background, etc. Another point of view is to consider the 'cat' as part of the person who is speaking or which he/she projects onto me. Yet another lets us think of said 'cat' as a feline quality which comes alive in the consulting room, probably generated by both patient and me, which it is my job to transform.

A colleague (Andrea Sabbadini, personal communication) has defined *'functional aggregate'* as 'a gestalt of verbal, emotional and bodily elements emerging in the analytic field' (see also Bezoari and Ferro 1992: 52). Ferro's *'affective hologram'* is described by Sabbadini (personal communication) as 'a three-dimensional description [representation] of affective dyadic interactions within the session'. In spite of my difficulty in grasping or remembering these definitions, let alone using them clinically myself, I find no difficulty in following Ferro's clinical material or in grasping his idea of what is happening in the analytic dyad and to its members in the clinical episodes he describes.

Ferro also makes a distinction between an analytic relationship based on transference/countertransference and what might be called a 'true' relationship. Ferro and Bezoari (1992: 59) say that: *'Transference* (including its necessary countertransference complement) [is a way of functioning] in which actuality is experienced in a stereotyped and repetitive way, where one member of the couple tends to force the other into fixed roles, predetermined by unconscious phantasies and induced by projective identifications.' Relationship, on the other hand, they define as 'a new intersubjective experience fully respectful of the partner's otherness, which can be continually symbolized' (Ferro and Bezoari 1992: 59). Conceptually I find this a useful distinction although in practice difficult to apply.

There are several ways in which I think Ferro does less than justice to current developments in Kleinian thought, and probably less than justice to developments in contemporary Freudian and ego-psychological thought as well. (My own edited book *Melanie Klein Today* vols 1 and 2 (1988) and Roy Schafer's more recent (1997) *The Contemporary Kleinians of London* give an overall view of much of the current Kleinian approach.) In the case of current Kleinian thought: all the Kleinians I know use the idea that the analyst is influenced emotionally by the patient's projections, and think that the analyst's use of his capacity for containment and transformation, together with careful observation and respect for the patient's material, is exceedingly important in the development of an analysis. 'Decoding meaning', as Ferro puts it, certainly has a place too, but there is increasing emphasis on the object of analytic study being the transference/countertransference relation-ship. This trend was already being developed by Klein herself, for her way of analysing patients as shown in *Envy and Gratitude* (1957) is rather different from her way of analysing Richard in 1941 (*Narrative of a Child Analysis*, 1961). There has been a gradual change by some Kleinian analysts in the direction of what I call 'descriptive' interpretations (Spillius 1994) and what John Steiner calls 'analyst-centred' interpretations, especially when patients are not able to accept responsibility for their thoughts and feelings (Steiner 1993). It is Ferro's idea that for Kleinian analysts the goal of analysis is to 'achieve' the depressive position, but it is many years since I have heard any colleague use that definition. One is more likely now to hear Kleinians speak of particular types of fluctuation between PS and D, or of withdrawal of projections from objects or greater flexibility in the use of defences. It is clear, however, that for most Kleinian analysts the point of the work is to understand the *patient* better, rather than to understand the analyst–patient relationship as an end in itself; understanding the analyst–patient relationship is a means to the end of understanding the patient.

I have mentioned above Ferro's dislike of 'saturated', closed interpretations which reveal a truth about the patient or about the analytic interaction regardless of whether the patient is able to accept the interpretation and regardless of whether it helps him to grow mentally. In Chapters 2 to 7 of the present book he gives innumerable examples of patients' symbolic statements indicating that Ferro should 'slow down', that his therapeutic zeal is too much for the patient, that he should let the patient develop at his own pace. (Actually in most cases he gives the patient's response but not his own preceding interpretation, so that it is difficult to know how the reader would feel about Ferro's interpretation.) Ferro is very much in agreement with Rosenfeld's idea (1986, 1987) that the analyst should allow the patient to idealize him without disillusioning him too soon and with Winnicott's statement (1971, especially pp. 62, 69) that the patient's self-discovery is far more important than the analyst's cleverness. The implication is that all three, Rosenfeld, Winnicott and Ferro, are critical of analysts who expect too much of the patient or, worse still, who treat the patient's criticisms of the analyst as based on envy or as an instance of the negative therapeutic reaction. When I questioned this implication and asked Ferro to expound his point of view further, this was his reply:

> I consider interpretations like cargo which has to be found a place on board a ship, but instead of a ship, there's a boat. We first must expand the boat (develop the [patient's] alpha function of the apparatus for thinking thoughts) before the weighty contents can be taken on board.

Nicely put, I thought, but nonetheless too categorical for my taste, just as an analyst who would always 'blame' his patient's envy or innate destructiveness would also be too categorical. It seems to me that once the analyst starts to think that the patient is usually 'right' and the analyst 'wrong', or that the analyst is usually 'right' and the patient 'wrong', something is seriously wrong with the analyst's curiosity and his capacity to think and feel impartially but with passion.

I think that perhaps Ferro has been attracted to Bion's thinking, especially his later formulations, and to the thinking of the Barangers about the bi-personal field in the hope that the intersubjective emphasis would counter any analyst's tendency towards dogmatism, analytic cleverness in decoding a patient's meanings, or moral pleasure in judgemental pronouncements. But a psychoanalytic theory is no protection against dogmatism. Is it not possible, for example, that the withholding of interpretations may be as arrogant and condescending as the aggressive display of interpretations designed to show the analyst's omniscience? It is, I believe, a matter of the analyst's personal character, integrity and sensitivity rather than his theory. More suitable theories need to be developed, of course, but they cannot control omnipotence and narcissism.

In this matter of who is 'right', the patient or the analyst, I think that Bion's thinking can help us. He was fond of saying that thoughts precede thinking, that thinking develops to deal with thoughts – a formulation that has puzzled many analysts, for one is used to thinking of thoughts as the product of thinking, which of course they also are. But Bion is drawing attention to the reciprocity of the process. If thoughts are the 'contained', and thinking is the 'container', then I think it is legitimate to expect that unfamiliar thoughts will stretch the container and that the recipient of them is likely to object, that he is likely to push the new thoughts away, to resent their alien origin, to define them as the arrogance or madness of the other, perhaps to conquer them by idealizing them and claiming them as his own, or to be overwhelmed by them into being unable to think. This happens to the analyst, of course, but it also happens to the patient. Ferro, I believe, thinks the analyst's thoughts should not exceed the capacity of the patient's container, or should be nicely calculated so as to be only a tiny bit ahead of the patient's containing capacity. I think that if thoughts were so limited, the container, whether it belongs to the analyst or the patient, would not develop. In my view we must take it for granted that thoughts are sometimes too big or too small for the container – or, of course, sometimes just wrong, inadequate – but better to err on the side of stretching the container rather than just fitting in with it.

But Ferro, whatever his theory – and his theory is interesting in its own right – has something of great value: clinical imagination. It is this that allows him access to his own unconscious and to that of his patients, a gift to treasure, and I believe that it is this gift that makes his book particularly valuable and the transmission of it particularly important. And I am glad that after much delay and many vicissitudes it will now be available to the English-speaking psychoanalytic world.

Elizabeth Bott Spillius

References

Baranger, M., Baranger, W. and Mom, J. (1983) 'Process and non-process in analytic work', *International Journal of Psychoanalysis* 64: 1–15.

Bezoari, M. and Ferro, A. (1989) 'Listening, interpretations and transformative functions in the analytic dialogue', *Rivista di Psicoanalisi* 35: 1014–1050.

Bion, W. (1959) 'Attacks on linking', in W. Bion, *Second Thoughts*, London: Heinemann, 93–110.

—— (1961) *Experiences in Groups*, London: Tavistock.

—— (1962a) 'A theory of thinking', in W. Bion, *Second Thoughts*, London: Heinemann, 93–109.

—— (1962b) *Learning from Experience*, London: Heinemann.

—— (1963) *Elements of Psychoanalysis*, London: Heinemann.

—— (1980) *Bion in New York and São Paulo*, Perth: Clunie Press.

Bléandonu, G. (1994) *Wilfred Bion: His Life and Works 1897–1979*, London: Free Association Books.

Britton, R. (1989) 'The missing link: parental sexuality in the Oedipus complex', in R. Britton, M. Feldman and E. O'Shaughnessy, *The Oedipus Complex Today*, London: Karnak House.

Ferro, A. and Bezoari, M. (1992) 'From a play between "parts" to transformation in the couple: psychoanalysis in a bipersonal field', in L. N. Momigliano and A. Robutti (eds) *Shared Experience: The Psychoanalytic Dialogue*, London: Karnac Books, 43–65.

Klein, M. (1935) 'A contribution to the psychogenesis of manic-depressive states', in *Writings*, vol. 4, *Love, Guilt and Reparation and Other Papers*, London: Hogarth Press and Institute of Psycho-Analysis (1975) 262–289.

—— (1940) 'Mourning and its relation to manic-depressive states', in *Writings*, vol. 1, *Love, Guilt and Reparation and Other Works*, London: Hogarth Press and Institute of Psycho-Analysis (1975), 344–369.

—— (1946) 'Notes on some schizoid mechanism', *International Journal of Psycho-Analysis* 27: 99–110.

—— (1957) 'Envy and gratitude', in *Writings*, vol. 3, *Envy and Gratitude and Other Works*, London: Hogarth Press and Institute of Psycho-Analysis (1975), 176–235.

—— (1958) Unpublished discussion in Melanie Klein Archive, Box 23, C72.

—— (1961) *Narrative of a Child Analysis. The Conduct of the Psycho-Analysis of Children as Seen in the Treatment of a Ten Year Old Boy*, London: Hogarth Press.

Lewin, K. (1935) *A Dynamic Theory of Personality*, New York: McGraw-Hill.

—— (1952) *Field Theory in Social Science*, D. Cartwright, ed., London: Tavistock.

Meltzer, D. (1978) *The Kleinian Development, Part III: The Clinical Significance of the Work of Bion*, Perth: Clunie Press.

Ogden, T. (1994) 'The concept of interpretive action', *Psychoanalytic Quarterly* 2(63): 219–245.

Rosenfeld, H. (1986) 'Transference–countertransference distortions and other problems in the analysis of traumatized patients', unpublished talk given to the Kleinian analysts of the British Psycho-Analytical Society, 30 April 1996.

—— (1987) *Impasse and Interpretation*, London: Routledge.

Sabbadini, A. (1997) Personal communication.

Schafer, R. (ed.) (1997) *The Contemporary Kleinians of London*, Madison CO: International Universities Press.

Spillius, E. Bott, (ed.) (1988) *Melanie Klein Today*, vol. 1, *Mainly Theory*, vol. 2, *Mainly Practice*, London: Routledge.

—— (1994) 'Developments in Kleinian thought: overview and personal view', *Psychoanalytic Inquiry* 14: 324–364.

Steiner, J. (1993) *Psychic Retreats: Pathological Organizations in Psychotic, Neurotic and Borderline Patients*, London: Routledge.

Winnicott, D. W. (1971) *Therapeutic Consultations in Child Psychiatry*, London: Hogarth and the Institute of Psycho-Analysis.

1

A review of the theoretical models

Many authors (Money-Kyrle 1968; Meltzer 1978; De Bianchedi 1991) have suggested simplifying adult psychoanalysis down to three fundamental models: the Freudian, the Kleinian, and a third model inspired by Wilfred Bion. In my view this tripartite division is equally valid for the analysis of children.

I am also of the belief that while other figures have made extremely important contributions to the advancement of this field, none has produced a truly unified model; rather, their work appears as a sort of 'variation on a theme'. Some have undergone complex evolutionary transformations. Herbert Rosenfeld's ideas and clinical approach changed considerably in his forty years of psychoanalytic practice. Meltzer started off from a strictly Kleinian stance but in recent years has adopted and given an original turn to some of the more radical elements in Bion.

Furthermore, I do not feel that there is anything particularly specific to the analysis of children (Ferro 1997) which would lead one to suppose that there are writers and problems specific to the analysis of adults and writers and problems specific to the analysis of children. In my view there is only one psychoanalysis, with varying clinical situations in which a 'realization'[1] must be found, using different models, and perhaps with different objects. However, stressing the differences confirms how each analytic encounter is unique and unrepeatable.

I lay no claim to objectivity or thoroughness in the few points I shall make in characterizing these models. I shall simply explain what place they have for me, and how I have experienced them in my work.

But before embarking on a review of the various models of psychoanalysis, let me point out that, talking schematically, a tripartite subdivision emerges in any case, if we seek to characterize the different models in terms of how they account for the characters or the facts related in the session (Ferro 1991; Bezoari and Ferro 1992). A brief review of these approaches,

1

which will be treated in greater detail in Chapter 5, may serve as an introduction to the issue.

According to one model of listening, the characters of the session are understood primarily as knots in a network of historical, factual relationships. Related facts, in this case, are occasions for the expression of feelings, conflict and emotional strategies, which are always connected with those characters. Alternatively, these facts, though considered present and real within the intrapsychic dynamics, may almost acquire an 'autonomous' existence. This, after all, is what we find in literary studies on character prior to the entrance on stage of Vladimir Propp.

In the second model (which is expounded most clearly by Klein and her followers) the characters are knots in a network of intrapsychic relationships. Related facts are ultimately a way to communicate the patient's inner reality in disguise, a reality, however, which is seen as already 'given'. It awaits an interpreter to clarify its functioning by discovering its root in the patient's unconscious phantasies. For example, it is extremely fruitful to study Klein's analysis of Richard and the way she perceives the characters that take shape in the session, or the way she interprets narrated facts, which are always traceable to the unconscious phantasies of the young patient.[2]

The third model – and we are now talking about Bion and the further development of his work – presents characters as knots in an interpersonal, or rather intergroup, narrative network, which emerge as 'holograms' of the current emotional interrelationship between analyst and patient. According to this view there are extremely primitive emotions, or better 'moods', at play in the session, which cannot yet be thought about. These moods are waiting for the analyst and the patient, using every possible means, to be in a position to receive them, to avoid being drowned by them, and to narrate them to each other.

The goal of the analytic couple (and of the 'group' that emerges from its work) is basically to communicate (generally, though not exclusively, through words) the emotions which pervade them. The characters are often 'created' then and there in the encounter and by the encounter of the two minds. The characters represent a way of sharing, narrating and transforming these primitive states of mind, helped by the psychoanalytical functions of the analyst's mind.[3] For example, in a famous passage in Bion (1962) in which 'ice-cream' (also frozen emotions) is transformed into the dramatic character 'I scream' – a cry that inevitably reminds us of Munch – it is desperation that here emerges as narrative expression.

Let us now return to the three models we began with. Characteristic of the Freudian model is the central importance of reference to the past attributed to the patient's communications. What the patient says is considered, with varying emphases, as having much to do with what he has actually experienced, whether in external reality or in psychic reality activated to some extent by external facts, as is the case of the well-known question of child seduction.

It is possible to investigate facts which in any case maintain a high level of historical truth. Facts can be reconstructed and revealed behind the opaque veil of repression. Various defence mechanisms work to obstruct the analyst's attempts at disclosure, and he is forced to remove them in order to arrive at a truth that must be revealed. Psychoanalysis becomes a sort of archaeology, though a 'living archaeology', to use Green's expression (1973).[4]

According to this model it is possible to know the patient, to examine his functioning and character independently. It is a model which, as the Barangers point out (1969), despite its elaboration as relation and dialogue, requires most of the concepts which make up its theoretical edifice to be formulated, as Freud thought, in monopersonal terms.

But let us get back to the model. Freud had brilliant insights: the method of free association instead of hypnosis and suggestion; the discovery of the intense bond created between patient and analyst; the transference, understood as a repetition of what cannot be remembered about early childhood; and the use of the interpretation as a way of making conscious what has been repressed, thus permitting the extension of the boundaries of consciousness.

It is well known that Freud continually revised his theoretical framework, adding new elements without ever completely eliminating the old ones. Certain concepts, however, remain central to his thought, such as 'trauma', 'instinct', 'infantile sexuality', and development in 'phases' (oral, anal, phallic, genital), each of which is accompanied by particular aspects of the functioning of the mind and personality.

Another remarkable theory concerns dreams. It is thanks to *Traumdeutung* and to Freud's rejection of more neurophysiological models that it is possible to explain the mind through the mind. Freud identifies specific ways in which the dream takes shape (the hallucinatory realization of wishes, condensation, censorship, displacement, symbolization, the day's residues) and the factors involved in the subsequent interpretation, which require the dreamer to help decode the dream. All this makes it possible to discover the latent meaning behind the overt text of the dream. This dream text must then be broken down into its component parts, so that it is possible for the patient freely to associate with each of its subunits, and the text must be connected to the patient's current life and childhood experiences.

One of the key concepts in Freud's thought is that of repression.[5] In 1906 Freud wrote that through repression something mental was pushed out of reach while at the same time being retained. It is as though events had to be dug up, as in Pompeii, even though the work of excavation must first cross the territory of the emotional present of the therapy. This passage, in turn, makes buried facts the 'living materials of the narrative' (Petrella 1988). In any case the idea is maintained that there is a historical nucleus of truth belonging to the patient and knowable. This in itself is considered to be a healing factor.

The mental apparatus is now necessarily described as having a first topography (conscious, preconscious and unconscious) and a second topography (id, ego and super-ego).

Of course, the above outline is little more than a sketch. Indeed, it would be interesting to investigate the implications of this model for symbolism, defences, interpretation, transference, countertransference, and so on, but this is not the place to do so.

We cannot leave Freud, however, without quoting one of his clinical cases, which was for him (and for anyone dealing with child analysis) of crucial importance. I am, of course, referring to Little Hans (1909). This case was extremely significant for Freud, since it gave him the opportunity to check in real life all the theories about development, infantile sexuality, the Oedipus complex, and so on, that had been based on the analysis of adults and could now be studied *statu nascenti*. The case is important for us because it provides the first model of child analysis. It gives us access to the paraverbal language of a child (comparable to free association), such as drawing, dreams and phantasies, which lays the foundations for a technique of child analysis.

As the reader will recall, we are dealing with a phobia about horses which Hans suddenly developed. Hans is not analysed directly but rather through his father, who does with Freud what today would be called supervision. Freud finds in Hans confirmation of the existence of infantile neurosis. He identifies as traumatic events the anxiety of castration (the mother's threats that the doctor would cut off his genitals if he kept on touching them), the birth of his sister Hanna (or rather, how he was lied to on that occasion, in open contradiction to what he himself perceived), the difficulties connected with evacuation and, finally, the imprecise description of the differences between the sexes.

Aberastury (1981) emphasizes that this list must be extended to include the trauma of the tonsillectomy, which she finds gave rise to the particular phobia about the colour of the 'white' horse, linked with the doctor's smock, like the fear that his fingers would be bitten ('the fingers of the doctor that operated on him'; the 'fingers of masturbation'). She also asserts that if sex had been adequately explained it might have prevented Hans's phobia. This is because the anxieties of castration were confirmed by the tonsillectomy, which showed that actual bodily mutilation was possible. Gradually, Freud showed the connections between the phobia, the Oedipal process, the reality of sexual instincts, the castration complex, and so on. Hans ingeniously proposes to keep his mother for himself, while offering his grandmother to his father in exchange, hoping that in this way everyone would be satisfied. As Hans's conflicts and fears become clear and manifest, the phobia finally disappears.

4

Even after many rereadings, this case continues to be surprising and fascinating, especially when it shows us Freud at work, with extraordinary delicacy, in the only direct encounter he describes with his young patient.

The father, who is often described by Freud as excessive and even intrusive, appears to be over-realistic. He frequently invades the boy with questions and queries to the point where once, in the course of one of these interrogations, in response to the umpteenth question on what he is thinking about, Hans answers: 'raspberry syrup and a gun for shooting people dead with', as if to say: 'About a bit of sweetness, and about shooting at anybody who torments me like that.'

It would be too easy for us today to criticize the interpretations and explanations given to the child, easy not to grasp how Hans himself felt 'like a crumpled giraffe' because of the often unsolicited clarifications. But we must not forget that we are in the year 1908, at the dawn of psychoanalysis, and that it is already quite amazing that meaning and attention were given to the words, phantasies and dreams of a 5-year-old child.

It is also true that in the case described there is a forced attempt to find in Hans's words confirmation of what was being sought. But, after all, this was a unique opportunity to confirm the theoretical foundations of the new science. 'Does the Professor talk to God, as he can tell all that beforehand?', Hans asks his father in amazement after a meeting with Freud, who had explained certain aspects of the Oedipus complex to him.

Meltzer (1978), of course, says that today it would be unthinkable, without running grave risks, either to explore a child's mental life so directly or to stimulate his unconscious phantasies. Moreover, he stresses the difference between reconstructive work, on the one hand, that is work aimed at confirming the hypothesis of infantile neurosis, which was carried out with Hans and, on the other, what Klein did with her young patients, which was from the very beginning evolutionary, as it focused on the development of the child.

It goes without saying that there have been an almost infinite number of elaborations of this Freudian text. Many have sought new truths and points of view, occasionally bordering on 'deconstructionism', which recognizes all possible interpretations. Freud's greatness lies not only in his monumental theoretical and clinical work, but also in the fact that he left us a method for work and research (Tagliacozzo 1990) that can be used to understand mental phenomena, and this is true also for child analysis.

After Freud, the attempt to analyse children was continued by Hug-Hellmuth (1921), who did not, however, leave us a systematic statement of her working procedure using play. Then we get to Sophie Morgenstern, who worked at the Heuyer clinic in France. Morgenstern left us a book on child psychoanalysis (1937) which shows that she placed priority on drawings. Drawings, in fact, had become necessary for the treatment of a 10-year-old boy who was affected by mutism but drew a lot. The successful therapy encouraged her to continue in the same direction. Rambert (1938), in Switzerland, introduced marionettes representing typical characters (the mother, the aunt, the father, the doctor, etc.) and used them to animate stories.

Anna Freud (1946) and Melanie Klein (1932) were the first to publish methodological books presenting systematic techniques for the analysis of children. For Anna Freud a preparatory period must precede the analysis. She lays stress on the use of dreams, daytime phantasies and drawings, while limiting that of play. We shall see how Melanie Klein's introduction of play in the analytic situation marked a revolutionary turning point in child analysis.

Before discussing this second model, I would like to mention a few of Anna Freud's attitudes and theoretical positions which, as we will see, are notably different from those of Klein, although they have subsequently undergone considerable reworking and modification (Aberastury 1981).

Anna Freud held that children do not have the capacity for transference, since they have not yet dissolved their primary external ties. Consequently, there can be no second version, if the first has not yet been exhausted. Children, in her view, need a preparatory period before they will accept therapy. They must have a positive environment, and negative situations that arise must be faced and resolved with non-analytic means. A constant pedagogical commitment is required of the analyst, since children have an immature super-ego. Free associations could not be replaced by play, or better, free play corresponds to free associations, whereas play in the consulting room is comparable to resistance against the continual interruptions and changes which the child faces.

Later Anna Freud was to give up the preparatory phase and placed the child directly in the analytic situation, but she remained firm on many other aspects of her theory. It is not my intention here to go into Anna Freud's many dynamic contributions, among which I should mention her insights into the defence mechanisms of the ego, that remain fundamental for the whole of psychoanalysis.

It is with Melanie Klein that we encounter a true revolution and the full, exhaustive formulation of a model of child analysis. But when we speak of Klein it is impossible to limit our attention to children, given the overall importance of her model for all psychoanalysis.

With Klein it becomes entirely possible to construct genuine child analysis, free of pedagogical aims, thanks to the brilliant introduction of play material (see Chapter 3) and to the equally ingenious intuition that the child continually performs an activity of personification (1929) by using toys in the session. This activity is in every way comparable to free association.

By listening to children Klein recognized how important the inner bodily 'spaces' are to them, both their mother's and their own. This discovery led to a revolution in the conceptualization of the geography of the mind (Meltzer 1979). The mind becomes a 'place' where things exist and happen. It is this predominantly visual image that gives rise to a 'theatrical' model of the mind, a model which aims to describe events as they occur inside these inner spaces rather than to reconstruct historical events, as in the Freudian model.[6] Transference now becomes the visible situation par excellence and the only one we can be sure about. The present of the patient–analyst relationship is clarified by understanding projective identifications, which in turn enriches our understanding of the countertransference. At the same time Klein is extremely attentive to the facts of the patient's external life, although she considers communications concerning external reality as connected to the unconscious phantasies underlying them.

Klein, then, lays far more emphasis than Freud on the functioning of the *inner world* and on the mental facts that occur in it. All psychic life is dominated by the activity of phantasies, that is, by the interplay between unconscious phantasies and the defences connected with them. We find derivatives of Freud's 'phases' in Klein's formulation of the paranoid–schizoid and depressive positions. Originally she considered these as following a chronological sequence, that is, as characterizing the evolutionary 'stages' of mental development. Later, she came to understand them as positions, each with its own characteristic combination of anxieties and defences. (Bion conceived the two positions as being in constant oscillation one with the other, joined schematically with a bi-directional arrow: PS$\longleftrightarrow$D. In Bion's view, this equilibrium characterizes the entire mental life of each individual.)

Primitive anxieties play a major role in Klein's model, such as those stemming from aggression, the death instinct, destructiveness, sadism, greed, envy, and the phantasied revenge of the attacked object. A good experience with the real external object, aided by the interpretations, gradually makes it possible to metabolize these anxieties and narrow the gap between the world of unconscious phantasies and that of external reality. The most primitive phantasies, the positives ones and especially the negative, must be immediately taken on and, above all, interpreted in the transference. Otherwise, the idealization or persecution will be directed at persons outside the analysis, with serious risks of acting out (Aberastury 1981).

It is perfectly understandable that Klein should give absolute priority to the meaning of communications and that the vertex should be the meaning of the transference in the present, as the analysis of Richard illustrates. On the one hand, interpretation facilitates contact with this inner world, with its distortions, misunderstandings, blindness, attacks, etc. On the other hand, it makes it possible to contact the most primitive bodily phantasies and to metabolize the underlying anxiety aroused by the death instinct by helping the patient to 'feel understood and relieved' (Lussana 1983).

Seen from this point of view, the analyst's job seems to me like that of a 'UN envoy' who negotiates the patient's relationship with the phantasies of his inner world. The patient distorts, attacks, splits, and projects; the analyst takes on these phantasies and makes the patient aware of the operations he is carrying out. Essentially, his job is to show the patient the gap between his way of functioning and external reality, and it is the analyst who mediates that reality.

Some extremely interesting elaborations on this model have been advanced (Corti 1981; Bott Spillius 1983, 1994; Bléandonu 1985; De Simone Gaburri and Fornari 1988; Joseph 1989; Lichtmann 1990).

1   Greater importance is given to internal reality, considered to be just as 'real' as the external one (and this explains the need to specify which reality one is talking about, whether external or internal).
2   Each individual is recognized as having an internal space where 'the facts of unconscious phantasies' actually occur.
3   Conflicts are backdated (in particular the Oedipus and the formation of the super-ego, whose violence and sadism are underlined), and attention is addressed to the most primitive anxieties, linked to experiences with the breast and other part-objects.
4   The most important contribution of all, so much so that it has become adopted by psychoanalysis generally, even those who are not Kleinian, is the description of *projective identification* as a mechanism serving to free the mind of anxieties (or parts), evacuating them outwards and, sometimes, into someone else who becomes the receptor of this process.[7]

Klein herself seems to have been somewhat alarmed at the profound implications of her intuition about projective identification. She advised analysts to be cautious in their use of countertransference (essentially the radar apparatus designed to intercept projective identifications). Careful attention, she stressed, should be paid to the interpretation of what the analyst observes in the patient. Indeed, she even produced, though piecemeal, what might be considered a *manifesto of her own way of observing* (see Chapter 3).

In this model, it seems to me, the patient is seen and described in 'his' way of functioning with us as he thinks we are.[8]

The analyst interprets in the present (then backdating in the patient's history and shifting to the reality outside the analysis) a transference relationship, understood as the outward projection of the patient's phantasies and internal ways of functioning. He interprets anxieties and defences. The neutrality of the analyst remains a firm principle (Saraval 1985). If this neutrality is occasionally lost, due to the patient's violent, evacuative projective identifications, it must be regained as soon as possible.

For Klein, projective identification is a factor of disturbance, as countertransference was for Freud. This disturbance has to be eliminated, for it indicates that something is not working the way it is supposed to. Consequently, violent projective identifications are not considered in relation to the fragility of the container or to its capacity to take on such projective identifications and transform them. For present-day Kleinians, thanks to general adoption of Bion's elaborations of Klein's concept, projective identification is now sometimes a disturbance, sometimes communicative, etc.

The analyst becomes the screen onto which the patient's most primitive unconscious phantasies are projected, and the answers which the patient provides to the interpretations are considered as further unconscious phantasies and as proof of the distortions met by the reception of the interpretation (Joseph 1984).

I should stress that the cornerstone of this model is the *projection of what the patient says* in the present of the transference (understood as the externalization of what happens in the inner world).

There are, to my mind, two lines of development on the Kleinian model. One lays stress on the underlying bodily phantasy. The other focuses more on the description of the qualities of the observed fact in terms of mental functioning, but this fact is always considered as reflecting the functioning of the patient's inner world, albeit in the 'true fiction' of the transference. The way of interpreting anal masturbation (Meltzer 1965) covers the entire range of possibilities from the visual description of the event to the interpretation of the psychic characteristics accompanying it.

In later reworkings of the Kleinian model there are certain points that remain absolutely central, in my opinion. One is that successful fluctuation between depressive[9] and paranoid-schizoid features guarantees mental health and, consequently, the prevalence of neurotic mechanisms over psychotic ones.

An interpretation referring to deep material chosen on the basis of its urgency is an *interpretation of transference* concerning the *present* of the relationship and what is 'outside and in the past'.

Segal (1979), in defining the characteristics of Kleinian analysis, adds the *rigour of the setting*, which serves to allow the deepest phantasies to manifest themselves without contamination, and the *capacity for attention* to all the ways in which, including projective identification, the patient may try to 'influence' the analyst's mind.

Another cornerstone of the Kleinian model is the concept of *unconscious phantasy*. Isaacs (1948), in her thorough description of the notion, defines it as the mental expression of instincts, instincts that can be perceived only by their mental representative. As long as the pleasure–pain principle is dominant, the phantasies are omnipotent and there is no distinction between the experiences of external reality and those of phantasy. In the mind of a breast-fed baby, the desire to eat becomes the omnipotent phantasy of having incorporated the nourishing ideal breast, whereas the desire to destroy becomes the omnipotent phantasy of having destroyed the breast and of being persecuted by it.[10] The omnipotence of phantasies is never total, however, since it is tempered by the experience of external reality.

For a more detailed treatment of the most important developments in Kleinian analysis, the reader is referred to Gaburri and Ferro (1988). I should mention, however, a few collective publications that give a full presentation of the Kleinian school. One is *Developments in Psychoanalysis*, published in 1952 by Klein and her closest collaborators. This volume completes the Kleinian model from a theoretical point of view. Another is *New Directions in Psychoanalysis* (1955) which bears witness to the conceptual depth of the model, its clinical fecundity and its applicability to other spheres of knowledge. A third is *Melanie Klein Today* (1988) edited by E. Bott Spillius. Last, the book by Roy Schafer (1997) entitled *The Contemporary Kleinians of London*.

The main areas of Klein's clinical work – the analysis of children and the analysis of severe borderline patients – come together to contribute both to a greater understanding of the analysis of 'neurotic' patients (making it possible to reveal basic underlying anxieties) and also to an extension of the clinical applicability of analysis to groups of patients and areas of patients previously considered as unreachable.

This change of vertex with respect to traditional patients was to have considerable influence on the definition of new models in the classification of diseases and in metapsychology. Moreover, the extension of the concept of analysability paved the way for new models of the mind.

The continual interchange between Klein and her pupils, and among her pupils themselves (as though a fabric were being woven by many hands), constituted a genuine conceptual revolution in the panorama of psychoanalysis. It affected not only clinical practice but also numerous other disciplines, ranging from aesthetics (Segal), to political philosophy (Money-Kyrle), groups (Bion), politics and war (Fornari), and social and institutional life (Elliot Jaques, Menzies-Lyth, and Salzberger-Wittemberg).

It should be stressed that the very fecundity of the Kleinian model permitted concepts originating within it to be used by analysts who do not consider themselves Kleinian. Indeed, some of these concepts are now common to the entire psychoanalytic movement. This is true above all of projective identification (Ogden 1979).

We have now arrived at the third model: Wilfred Bion's. Although some (Bott Spillius 1983 and Bléandonu 1985) have sought to treat Bion's work as an evolution of Klein's, Bion, in my view, especially in his later work, represents a sharp break with the Kleinian model, just as Klein marked a break with Freud.

The least common denominator of all Bion's work can be identified, I believe, in the fundamentally different status he assigns to the *mental life of the*

analyst. Bion rewrites metapsychology in such a way as to include the observational experience of the analyst in the field of observation (Vergine 1991).
Since Bion entered the scene, it has become necessary to take into account
the continuous interactivity between analyst and patient whenever we assess
the progress and results of an analytic experience (Bordi 1990).

These developments have received criticism, it should be noted, from
those who 'seek to confine psychoanalytic activity to what is still
comprehensible of the Freudian model of 1924, or to what in any case can
be justified and given theoretical expression in Freud's work' (Di Chiara
1991).

This would be the place for a brief presentation of Bion's thought and of
the theory and technique his model entails. But I will refer the enquiring
reader once again to Gaburri and Ferro (1988), in which a discussion will be
found of the implications of Bion's thought on how we can conceive symbolism, projective identification, the interpretation and interpretive language.
The article also treats the chronological progression of his works and shows
the gradual emergence of a new model of the mind, of thought and of mental disturbances.

General annotated synopses of Bion like that published by Grinberg *et al.*
(1972) or the more recent one by Neri *et al.* (1987) are also recommended.
Needless to say, there is no substitute for Bion's own writings, in particular
the seminars, which constitute an endless source of learning and inspiration.
Though I hope that many of Bion's ideas will become clear in the following chapters, as much of the clinical material draws inspiration from his
work, or at least this is my intention.

There is one point, however, that requires mention and constitutes what
I consider to be the leitmotif of all of Bion's work. I am referring to the
*entirely new way in which the analyst's mind, his functioning and his dysfunctions
enter the field*. In Bion's view, the analyst is present with all the weight of his
mental life. Projective identifications are not merely the patient's evacuative,
disturbing operations into the analyst. They are also a perfectly normal way
for human minds to communicate. It follows, then, that they are reciprocal
and intersecting.

The 'story' that is developed will be entirely new and 'couple specific', in
terms both of its creative evolution and its healing and mutilating effects. It
is not the interpretive activity of decodification that counts. What is important is the transformation of the patient's projective identifications. This is a
task for the the analyst, who must be aware that he plays an active role in
determining the facts. The very presence of the analyst, as observer, is influ-
ential, but even more so are his defensive structures and relative projective
identifications.

The other half of the story of the analysis will be scripted by the analyst's
defences, his receptivity or non-receptivity to the patient's projective

identifications and his capacity to modify, through his own mental functioning, what Bion calls the 'beta-elements' arriving from the patient (as well as his own).

I should stress that Bion is concerned not so much with the content of thought as with the mental apparatus that makes thinking possible. This turns every approach to the patient (and to the psychotic parts of every patient) upside down. What is important, then, is not work on repression (Freud) or splitting (Klein). Rather, we must go back to the source: we must work on a 'place' where thoughts can be thought. In other words, we must work on the container before dealing with the contents.

The difference is illustrated vividly in Gaburri (1992). If Freud worked on what had been erased from a magic writing pad, Bion raises the question of how the drawing board or pad itself could be fixed or built. In other words, he was interested in the instrument for dealing with thoughts.

This operation is above all emotional and affective, the sort that takes place in the ($\female$ $\male$) child–mother relationship through reverie. This is what happens when we are in unison with the patient, which means not searching for objective or historical truths but rather being on the same affective wavelength with him. It means offering him a model of mental relationship that is capable of being introjected and does not require the acquisition of data but rather of 'qualities' (patience, passion, etc.) (Gaburri and Ferro 1988; Di Chiara 1990).

We do not find in Bion the idea that there is something to discover or to interpret. Rather, there is something that must be built up in the relationship, with the help of that 'unison' which makes it possible to expand the mind and the capacity to think, which is necessary for doing something about and with the thoughts.

As regards technique, De Bianchedi (1991) stresses that Bion proposes an attitude without memory and without desire: a disciplined attitude in which the capacity to tolerate the unknown is connected to a faith in *something* that develops through the emotional contact with the patient, and a faith that this *something* can be expressed in words, making possible a drastic change in the patient. This drastic change, moreover, implies a sudden leap in mental growth (Corrao 1981).

Clearly, Bion stands on Klein's shoulders, and the two models can be considered as oscillating one with the other. Each, in fact, allows us to approach certain truths from precise vertices. Let me stress, however, the profound differences between the two models, a point made in Gaburri and Ferro (1988). These differences lie not only in the theoretical frameworks, but also in the operative techniques of the two models. It is not my intention to detract from the value of Klein's model. Indeed, without Klein's discoveries there would be no psychoanalysis of children, nor of psychotics, nor of all those more primitive states of mind with which we have become accustomed to dealing. Rather, I hope to show that with Bion we achieve a break with the earlier model and arrive at the elaboration of a new, coherent one that paves the way, in the opinion of many of us, for the future of all psychoanalysis.

In the *Kleinian model* the analyst is placed in a privileged position with respect to the patient, and he always has a solid theory to refer to. In the *Bionian model*,[11] in constrast, the analyst is aware that in the analytic session we are dealing with two dangerous, ferocious animals (Bion 1978, 1980) whose powerful emotional natures are quite distant from civilizing forces.

In the first of these models the analyst tends to be anchored to the depressive position and helps the patient, who is not, gradually to approach this position. The patient's journey follows a sequence marked by relatively linear, defined and codified stages that progressively lead him to achieve mental health. In this view, the analyst presides over the unfolding of a process.[12]

In the second model, what counts is not so much what the analyst, or the analysand, can do but rather what the couple can do (Bion 1983). The analyst's role is like that of the officer on a battlefield. He has the same feelings of fear, anxiety and terror as his men (essentially, fluctuations between the paranoid–schizoid and the depressive positions of the analyst's mind in the session, PS←→D). At the same time, however, he must also command. He cannot avoid sharing these feelings (otherwise he is absent, far from the battlefield, as we will see shortly), but he must also be their master. He is in danger, just like the patient, and aware that thinking is a new function of living matter (Bion 1978, 1980). He is threatened by the catastrophic violence of the 'truth' of the mental facts he is called on to share. He is in danger, if he is willing to venture to where his patient is ('being in unison') by way of a group encounter of the two minds in the session. What in a group is a person or a character distributed in space (Bion 1983), in a mind becomes the condensation of a spatio–temporal grouping. What is at stake can no longer be a healing, as a point of arrival, but rather the awareness that even the analyst is a bad deal who can never be completely analysed and that sooner or later the analysis will have to end, after which all we can do is the best we can with what we are (Bion 1980).

In the first model the patient projects, distorts, attacks or adheres, and acts subtly in the transference. The analyst, in essence, is benevolently aware of all this, in part distanced, but also not responsible for what the patient says or does (assuming he sticks to clinical orthodoxy).

In the second, on the contrary, it is the patient who observes and communicates to the analyst how the latter relates to him (Bion 1983; Meltzer 1986a; Rosenfeld 1987), since the patient is considered the best colleague we could ever have (Bion 1978, 1983); but also because he describes the analyst as he moves away or shows that he cannot tolerate what he, the patient, says.

13

In a passage of extraordinary emotional pregnancy in the *Italian Seminars* (1983) Bion shows how earthshaking it is to recognize that we can become *mentally absent*, when we do not like what the patient is saying, and that the patient with a serious mental disorder always knows when the analyst has become mentally absent. If the patient says 'You have gone away', the analyst will be greatly tempted to give a rationalizing interpretation, alluding to the anxieties of separation for the weekend, or the end of the analysis, as it would be far more difficult to say quite simply: 'You feel that I'm not really paying attention.'

This raises the question of how much truth about the patient, and about himself, the analyst is able to tolerate, i.e. how much truth about 'that analyst' with 'that patient' at 'that moment'. The analyst becomes tired because he is constantly being observed by his patient as regards the quality and genuineness of his mental functioning. And this is the price he pays for being an analyst (Bion 1983). The patient functions as a sort of mirror, reflecting the analyst's distance. This mirror allows the analyst not only to make amends in the relationship but also to observe the things he did not want to hear or could not bear hearing, such as the emotions he could not tolerate and his own dark zones, shielded or covered with still painful scars. In this sense the mirror is not unlike a countertransference dream of the analyst (Barale and Ferro 1987).

In the Kleinian model there is basically a sort of fear of transgression (Gaburri 1982) and a prevailing need for a firm theory requiring linear development, but one that must be respected 'faithfully'. The model that derives from Bion, on the other hand, asks the analyst to be conscious of the risk he runs as he carries out a search that can be formulated in terms of a model only at a rather abstract level – precisely in order to avoid the creation of theoretical pigeonholes. One is also aware that working too close to one's own theory in the session can result in shallow mental functioning. The analyst risks simply performing a simultaneous translation of the patient's words into the corresponding equivalent of the theory he employs. The risk, in a word, is that of an 'adhesive identification' with the model and with the patient (Bick 1968; Meltzer 1975).

In the Bionian model we find that interpretation, however subtle, is no longer central. Emphasis is now laid on the bi-personal field (or, as Meltzer puts it, the 'group of two') of the analysis. What counts in this field is the fact that two minds are in relationship, the way they relate and the emotional facts that take place in the field. For example, the 'alphabetization' of beta elements takes place not only as a result of verbal interpretations but also because of the succession of verbal and emotional relationships between the members of the couple. Both members of the couple, it should be stressed, are involved in manoeuvres designed to protect themselves from the possibility that the impending danger might turn into nameless terror, and both are concerned with the growth of their minds. This growth is not measurable in terms of the quantity of acquisitions but as increased willingness to accept them (Gaburri and Ferro 1988).

A new relationship is formed. On the one hand, this relationship changes the earlier ways of relating. On the other, it stands beside them. This new relationship involves the mental functioning of the analyst, then and there, as he relates to the patient and how he interprets or does not interpret. It takes into account his capacity to change his own mental and interpretive organization and his willingness to give up making saturating, unambiguous interpretations. It follows that an active role is assigned to the patient, by allowing him, for example, to use his own meanings to fill in the gaps of an open-ended plot, such as that of 'narrative interpretations' ('What story are we to tell?', asks Bion 1987) or 'group-type interpretations'. These are the factors of the relationship that make it possible for the patient to function mentally in a new way.

Each clinical problem[13] will require its own vertex in view of the psychopathologies, reconstructions and precocious phantasies involved. The question can be addressed by paying attention to how the two minds function and approach each other in the session. For instance, in the case of homosexuality, whether male or female, it is important to realize what sort of coupling the two minds perform in the session. It may be homosexual, if of the unproductive ♂ ♂ type, with the analyst forcing interpretations on a patient unprepared or unwilling to receive them, or with the patient speaking to an unreceptive analyst. It could also be of the ♀ ♀ fusional type, which blurs distinctions and resists the penetration of words (and reciprocal projective identifications). In this case nothing productive, nothing with potential to transform happens in the session. Thoughts (or children in the primal scene) are not born, because the functioning of the two minds is not ♀ ♂. In this functioning the receptive analyst receives the patient's words and projective identifications, transforms them and gives them back to him at a 'temperature' and in a 'form' he can bear. The patient takes them in, adds further preconceptions or expectations to them and returns them once again to the analyst. This functioning implies a mental mode of pairing (or a primal scene) in which new thoughts are born, the fruit of a good reciprocal union, without jealousy, envy or at least the -K of both members having obstructed the fertile functioning of the mental couple.

Indeed, while writing to Fliess, Freud said that every sexual act was a process involving four people. We are dealing with 'a relationship . . . that implies both partners being simultaneously and reciprocally subject and object, active and passive', as Fornari (1975) puts it. What is new here is the way in which we consider the facts that emerge in the session: not as history repeating itself, nor as archaic phantasies, nor as allusions to the bodily or sexual spheres. Instead, such events are considered exclusively as an expression of the 'mental' – and the 'mental' is the only object we are interested in and can know through the analysis (Alvarez 1985) – and consequently as an expression of the here and now of the two minds functioning in the session.

This brief review of the three basic models of psychoanalysis would be incomplete without some mention of the more striking and significant developments which have emerged in recent years in Latin America. For the sake of brevity, I shall merely list some of the most important figures: Racker (studies on countertransference); Pichon-Riviere (work on operative groups and links between psychoanalysis and social psychology); Bleger (studies on the psychotic part of the personality and the agglutinated nucleus); Libermann (communication); Aberastury (child psychoanalysis); Etchegoyen (the theory of technique); Raskovski (the psychic life of the foetus and infanticide); Alvarez de Toledo (the analytic dialogue); Grinberg (projective counteridentification, guilt and depression and the pathologies of migration); Gear and Liendo (the application of the theory of communication and structuralism to the psychoanalysis of the couple and the family); Chiozza (psychosomatics); Cesio (hypochondria and psychosomatics); Badaracco (studies on dreams and the 'object that drives one crazy'), and others. These authors must be given credit for having brought together lines of thought deriving from Klein and current tendencies in French and North American psychoanalysis, thus giving rise to original, fertile insights which in recent years have had an increasing influence on the more interesting and dynamic developments in psychoanalysis today.

In conclusion, I would like to draw attention to two authors who elaborated a theoretical framework which has certain important elements in common with Bion and at the same time certain irreconcilable differences. I am referring to Willy and Madeleine Baranger (later joined by Mom) and their characterization of the analytic situation as a 'bi-personal field'.

Let us begin with the Barangers' key article (1969a), in which they merge the concept of the field (borrowed from phenomenology, especially Merleau-Ponty) with the key concepts of Kleinian psychoanalysis. In this paper they describe the analytic situation as that of a bi-personal field in which only the *unconscious phantasy of the couple* can be known. The structure of this field is determined by the two mental lives and by criss–cross projective identifications passing back and forth between analyst and patient. It is expected, of course, that there will be a greater flow of projective identifications passing from the patient to the analyst. Periodically, and physiologically, the accumulation of criss-crossing projective identifications creates pockets of 'resistance' in the couple (not in the patient!). These zones require special attention on the part of the analyst, who with his *second glance* must recognize and interpret such blind spots, as they are an obstacle to analytic progress. The Barangers call these pockets of resistance 'bastions' (Baranger and Baranger 1969a,b; Baranger *et al.* 1983).

The vitality of this concept is enormously important, in my view. First, it allows us to overcome the notion that unconscious phantasies are pertinent only to the patient. Second, and more importantly, it recognizes the analyst's mental functioning as being 'in action', structured by the patient's functioning, but also structuring the functioning of the patient. The analyst must continually immerse himself; he is involved, captured by the projective identifications in the field. He almost reaches the point of assuming a role (Gear *et al.* 1976), only to use his second glance to regain awareness and interpret the projective identifications to the patient.

We are not far from some of Bion's ideas. An example is Bion's maxim that the patient always knows what his analyst is thinking and how his mind is functioning, and that the patient is the analyst's best colleague. We must continually receive his points of view on us and on the facts of the analysis, as this is the best way to reach him and to be in unison with him.

But there is a profound difference. It is true that in the Barangers' work the two mental lives (the analyst's and the patient's) appear to a certain extent closely intertwined and united in forming the unconscious phantasies of the couple. However, we still have 'strong' interpretations. The analyst interprets the unconscious phantasy of the couple as it emerges, in order to overcome the bastion and to put the couple back on the road until it encounters the next bastion, and so on. Not only do we have what can be called without hesitation a strong interpretation coming from the analyst, or more precisely from his second glance, but we also have the notion that, session after session, or even many times within the same session, it is always possible to know the moment when anxiety emerges and then to communicate it (Baranger *et al.* 1983).

With Bion, such certainties are abandoned. Instead, we find a preference for open-ended ('unsaturated') interpretations (see the notion of 'weak interpretations' described in Bezoari and Ferro 1989) and the continual creation – as opposed to the decoding – of new meanings. We find an awareness of what processes and transformations are necessary for the moment when anxiety emerges to be grasped. Bion is also sensitive to the time it may take before interpretations can be given, perhaps six days or six months later (Bion 1987).

The concept of the 'field' is more extensive than that of the relationship. It encompasses the entire analytic relationship, including the setting and the rules, and provides a broader range of vision than the notion of the relationship can offer. Many things can be thought of in advance, before they are actually transmitted in the relationship. We are dealing with a sort of middle ground which may give rise to scenes and characters that would otherwise remain trapped in a premature elucidation of relational movements (Manfredi Turillazzi and Ferro 1990). Corrao (1986) defined the field 'as a function whose value depends on its position in space and time: it is a system

17

with an infinite number of degrees of freedom, and these degrees have an infinite number of possible values which the system takes on at every point in space and every moment in time'.

Bion's notion of 'unsaturated' interpretations, Klein's 'personification of split-off parts', the Barangers' 'field' conceived as the time and place of the encounter between the analyst's and the patient's projective identifications, the focusing on the minute details of the dialogue in the session (Liebermann and Nissim), the attention to the creation, development and transformation of characters and narrations (Gaburri and Di Chiara); these are some of the guiding principles that have inspired much of the work that lies behind the pages that follow.

When we speak of different models, each having its own truth (or rather, its own approach to the truth), it becomes difficult to grasp similarities and differences. It would certainly be interesting to investigate the connections between the interplay of criss-crossing projective identifications in the session (Baranger), the split-off parts of the mind in the session (Klein and Rosenfeld), the personifications of such parts (Klein and Bion), the role of reciprocal internal groups (Meltzer) and basic assumptions (Bion) in relation to bastions (Baranger). But I feel that overdoing it with the microscope and the scalpel would strip these concepts of that sheen of open-endedness which makes their further development possible.

A special place should be reserved for Winnicott, for the originality, insight and clarity of his contributions. Among the many, we should recall the transitional object and area, the concepts of holding, of the mother with sufficient capacity and of true and false self. But if we went into these points, we would be likely to start reflecting on the models, whereas the intention was to present a simple introduction to the theory of the technique of the analyst at work.

2

Drawings

We are indebted to Balconi and Del Carlo Giannini (1987) for their book containing a wealth of detail on children's drawings. I refer the reader to that volume, both for the historical background it provides and for the in-depth discussion of how attention to drawing and the evolution of therapeutic relationships intertwine and develop in the clinical cases described.

I would like to recall, however, a few milestones in the study of drawings in child analysis. The first of these is little Hans's addition to his father's picture of a giraffe (Freud 1908), that is, the giraffe's 'widdler'. Then there are the drawings from Klein's analysis of Richard in 1941 (Klein 1961). More recently we have the extraordinary book on 'Squiggles' by Winnicott (1971a) which confirms, *ante literam*, both the characteristics of the bi-personal field and the creation of microstories shared with very young patients.

In this chapter, I will not consider all those works which regard the drawing as a test, nor those which adopt highly formalized approaches, as the subject has already been dealt with exhaustively (Dolto 1948; Widlocher 1965; Widlocher and Engelhart 1975). Indeed, leaving aside the more formalized interpretive schemes, there are still many ways of considering a drawing.

One way might be to regard the drawing as a representation of the types of relationship present in the child's emotional world, to a certain extent connected with external reality. This approach is often adopted in the interpretation of family drawings.

Figure 2.1 is the drawing of a twin, Franca, just separated from her sister, who is going to go to a different class at school. In her sister's place there is a spot, a sort of hole. The same drawing, if considered within the context of an analytic session, could indicate that there is a 'hole in understanding', a blind spot, something waiting to be thought about (Tagliacozzo 1982).

In a nearly identical drawing (Figure 2.2) made by Franca's sister, Lisa, the same black spot seems to weigh down on the ground, making Lisa bounce up in the air. Within the context of a session this drawing might be

Figure 2.1

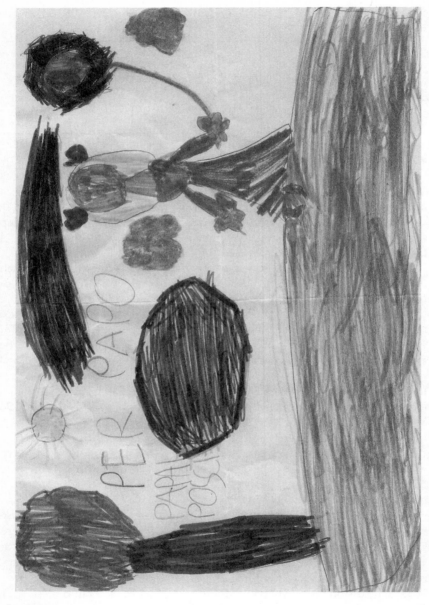

Figure 2.2

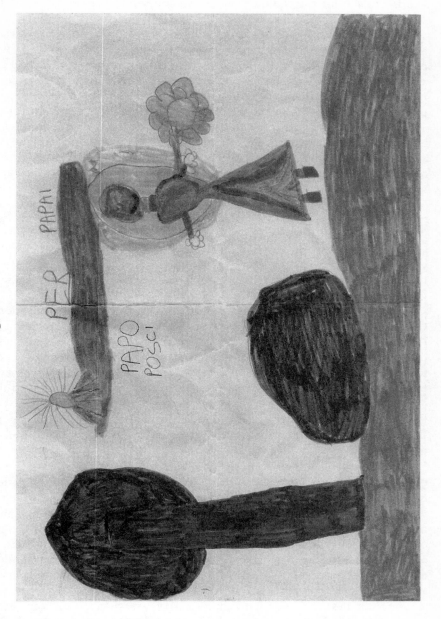

interpreted as representing the analyst's excessively forceful and weighty words which cause the child to lose contact and detach herself from the relational plane of communication.

Any interpretive approach to a drawing, then, depends on the perspective and the context. It is my view that within the analytic relationship (and I will consider drawings exclusively from this vertex) the drawing can be regarded as a sort of 'dream-like snapshot of the waking state' which photographs a relational, affective truth of the couple and of the field from an unknown point of view. However, what is still awaited is a narrative development. In other words, the drawing is *not there to be decoded*, not because this would not be possible, but we must ask ourselves what the point would be. Rather, it is a collection of ingredients for possible stories, a source for tales, a 'pre-text' requiring reverie and narration. It is like pushing the pause button on a video recorder and getting a frozen image from an ongoing film.

But let us step back a moment. As we said, the drawing can be considered as a sort of window into the child's internal world through which we can visualize what is happening following transferential movements in the here and now. It is Klein, of course, who has given us a complete outline of this way of considering drawings (and also games) in the analysis of children; and it is from this perspective that we should observe the technique she uses in interpreting Richard's drawings.

This approach to children's drawings has taken two different directions. One of these continues to lay stress on *unconscious phantasy*, with its references to body parts underlying the drawing. The same technique can be used in the interpretation of verbal material in which one can always look for and expose the *patient's* underlying unconscious phantasy. Unconscious phantasy is seen as something that pertains to the child as such, and to the child's phantasy world, which can be externalized on paper and projected in the transference. This interpretive mode has been further developed by considering the 'symbols' contained in the drawing as the structure, the web of the child's mental functioning.

Another approach focuses on the mentalization of the child's transference phantasies. It ignores reference to the body, since the object of interpretation is the type of mental functioning at work at a particular moment, which is understood, however, as the quality of the child's projection of phantasies into the therapist. The therapist remains substantially neutral, and the weight of her own mental activity does not enter the field which she shares in creating through the defences she activates and, especially, through her emotional receptiveness (Rosenfeld 1987) to the projective identifications arriving from the patient.

The therapist can use a drawing as she would a dream and elicit associations which she will think of as the *patient's* associations with the drawing. She will thus help the patient to verbalize, as completely as possible, what is already contained in the images of the picture but which await an interpreter.

These are ways of interpreting which, we might say with Todorov (1971), draw on a code which allows translation, producing the effect of melody and a parallel counter-melody.

While always keeping our debt to little Hans and Richard in mind, it is worth pointing out that there are other ways of considering drawings. I am thinking in particular of those which, with a certain Kleinian resonance, draw inspiration in part from the concept of the 'field' as defined by the Barangers with Mom (1969a, 1983) and by Corrao (1986). This implies that the analytic situation is conceived as a Gestalt which includes the analyst; and the analyst shares, with her own story, her internal world, her mental functioning and her defences, in the creation of this dynamic field which acquires structure through the interplay of projective identifications in accordance with the analytic contract. On the other hand these approaches are also influenced by Bion's recognition of the patient's ability to draw attention to the analyst's own mental functioning. Thus conceived, the drawing makes reference to the actual ways in which the analytic couple functions mentally in the here and now, to the dynamics of the bi-personal situation, and to the emotional forces of the field belonging to both members of the couple. The drawing is no longer considered only to be a reflection of the phantasies about the transference, but rather to be an authentic dream-like photograph of the mental functioning of the couple at a given moment, although taken from a particular and often as yet unknown perspective which we must share if we are to reach the patient on his own ground (Ferro 1994).

This approach makes it possible not only to recognize in the drawing how the couple's emotions evolve but also (once we have done away with the illusion that we can immediately find the point at which anxiety emerges) to construct, together with the patient, all the possible narrative developments.

As in the analysis of adults, weak interpretations (Bezoari and Ferro 1989), precisely because they are unsaturated, make the progressive formation of a shared meaning possible.

Drawings, then, are no longer static, in need of a code and a translation. They become animated like a sort of affective theatre, a theatre which generates sense and meaning (Meltzer 1984) in the course of the constructive development which the two minds will be able to promote.

From this point of view, the characters, the objects and the places of the drawing can been seen as holograms of the mental functioning of the couple, similar in this sense to the concept of 'functional aggregate', as we have called the visual development brought about by the narration of the mental functioning of the analytic couple in the session.

23

In my view, then, the drawing is connected to the mental functioning of the analytic couple at a given moment, that is, it is connected to a current problem. It appears as a 'bastion' (Baranger) which is also a beginning of the couple's transformative and creative resolution.

The patient's drawing

The drawing and construction of a story: Francesca

Ten-year-old Francesca, whose parents immediately strike me as 'fragile', has a strange symptom: she spends several hours a day screaming desperately, without stopping. She has had consultations and many diagnostic examinations, but to no avail. She has this problem only when she is at home, whereas in other environments her behaviour is appropriate and 'normal'. Neither she nor her parents can offer any explanation.

At her first meeting with me Francesca draws a picture (Figure 2.3). I feel rather uncertain in the face of all the possible meanings of the 'wood where there aren't any people' (as she calls it), inhabited by trees, wolves, snakes, fish and so on. I think of possible interpretations and wonder what use Francesca could make of them. None appears satisfactory.

In the meantime, I get a growing sense of uneasiness because I can't find the right words. I'm tempted to get out of the impasse by saying something, anything. Francesca seems to come to my aid by drawing another picture (Figure 2.4), which depicts a girl in profile, *without depth*. She is wearing lace and appears quite formal and composed.

But even – or perhaps even more so – with this drawing I can't make up my mind to step in. Thoughts come to mind about the two-dimensional quality of the drawing, about its lack of depth. I want to say something, even if it means drawing on my anxiety, my discouragement, my paralysis, which surely – I feel – have to do with Francesca, with her history, her symptom, her mental functioning. But *what* can I say to her, and *how* can I say it in such a way that it will be useful to her?

As my painful silence wears on (the length of which seemed to me to extend far beyond the few instants that actually passed), Francesca suddenly puts the second drawing next to the first: the 'two-dimensional girl' next to the 'wood without people'. At this point I get a sort of illumination and I ask Francesca excitedly: 'But what is a little girl doing all alone in a wood without people?' 'SHE'S SCREAMING!' is her stentorian reply. Then she begins to draw another girl (Figure 2.5), this time seen from the front. The figure has a three-dimensional appearance and intense eyes. The drawing remains incomplete because the session is over, but also because considerable work will be necessary before Francesca's anxieties can be expressed completely

Figure 2.3

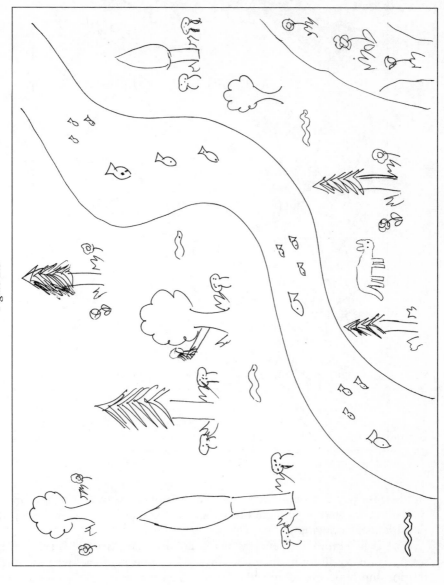

Figure 2.4

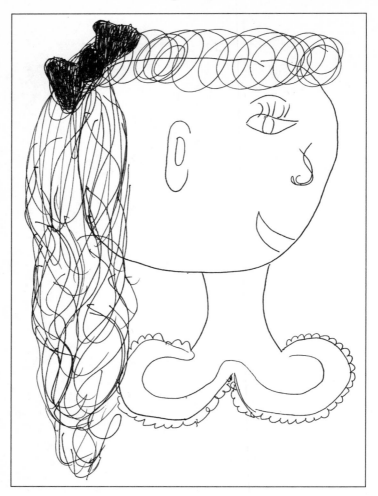

and before they can be expressed in words (note the absence of the mouth which she does not draw here but which in due time will find its own place in subsequent drawings).

This brief clinical sequence, which I cite from Bezoari and Ferro (1991c) seems to me to illustrate in simple form a few aspects of the dynamic inter-relationship between the affective and cognitive experiences which charac-terize the analytical field (Corrao 1988) and to which I would like to direct attention.

Figure 2.5

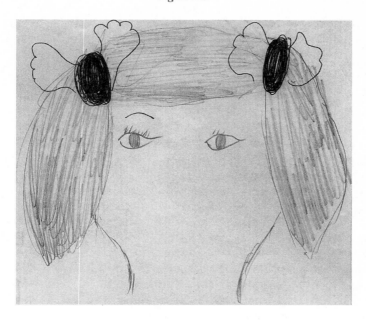

When I consider Francesca and her first drawing, I am immediately offered the possibility of locating the patient's message – the graphic and verbal elements of which appear to be well structured – in a universe of meaning which is familiar to me, thus allowing me to give Francesca a translation/ interpretation. But this seems adequate neither to my desire to come closer to the girl's point of view, nor to my responsibility towards her. (What would she do with a manual on botany and zoology explaining the contents of the wood?)

Once I loosen the ties to my theoretical referents, I begin to sense the risk of getting lost. 'Weak' models (and parents) expose us to the fear of thinking and finding ourselves *alone* in the wood, whereas 'strong' models would make us feel safe, but they would allow us to see in the wood only what the models themselves had already prefigured.

The second drawing increases my awareness of the contrast between the build-up of increasingly restless emotions and a formal thought mode unable to contain and express them. The drama of Francesca's 'double life' is gaining ground within me, in the time/space of the session.

But it is precisely this juxtaposition, in tune with the girl's gesture of putting the two drawings side by side, that sets in motion a new organization of the experiential field. In the 'wood without people' another encounter has taken place, and we are no longer alone. The lost and nameless emotions, which before could only be screamed out, are now included in a shared space and transformed into an experience which we can begin to relate: a microstory takes shape in the here and now, making it possible, once combined with the microstories of subsequent sessions, to construct a shared 'story'. This story will tell about, and render thinkable and communicable, emotions and affects which were previously either silent or uncontainably 'screamed out' in disorganized form, devoid of a shared meaning.

The construction of affective sense: Marco

Marco is an 8-year-old boy. At our first meeting he draws a black and white picture (Figure 2.6), completely lacking colour, recalling Marco's 'dull' appearance with his grey suit. I feel a sense of loss. I am tempted by the 'devouring oral quality' of the shark and by other possible 'symbolic' meanings, but am blocked by the idea that such interpretations would only serve to increase my feeling of disorientation.

Guided by this awkward sense of being 'lost', I think that finding each other, establishing contact, would already be something worthwhile, so I say that the drawing seems to me appropriate to our situation, that we do not actually know very much about each other, and that very little of the drawing appears above the surface of the water while all the rest is submerged, just like the things we have to discover.

In answer to my comment he adds the diver and the ship. I say that an adventure is unfolding with discoveries in store, and I note, as I look at the ship, that 'maybe there's a treasure in there', consciously thinking of something hidden inside it.

Marco shows that he has perceived the affective implication of what I have said. Suddenly he becomes excited and starts colouring in all the animals. Then he draws a traffic light, with alternating red and green lights, which he uses to indicate whether the suggestions I make are right or wrong.

I'm amazed, not only by the sudden transformation of our black and white adventure film into technicolor, but also by the shifting of the vertex it suggests with regard to the shark: there is something that is trying to get out, trying to free itself from the fish's jaws.

I should stress that there is no decoding of the meaning *of the drawing*. Rather, an affective-emotional story is set in motion by unleashing emotions and feelings in the couple through the projective identifications that create 'the treasure' which comes to life in the session.

What is important is not to make needs explicit but, as Bion puts it, the 'realization' of the 'preconceptions' waiting to be experienced in the current situation of the relationship. All this can take place if a significant, unique,

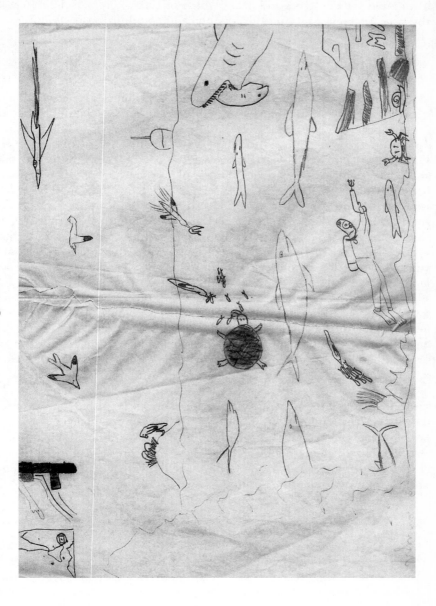

Figure 2.6

unrepeatable emotional experience is created that draws vitality from the mental work (reverie) which occurs within the couple. This can come about if we leave aside schemes and codes which might merely indicate the availability of 'instruments', but not of mental and emotional spaces.

The drawing as a starting point for narrative: Mariella

Mariella is 8 years old. She shows deep signs of a trauma. Her mother had a stroke that paralysed her and subsequently made her violent, impulsive and uncontrollable, to the point where it became necessary for her to separate from both her husband and daughter.

At our first meeting Mariella appears to be vigorous, strong and self-assured. Her father's new partner and her older sister have, it seems, replaced her mother. She is also doing well at school. She does a drawing (Figure 2.7) which strikes me for its lack of grace. I am reminded of the cow Clarabella, and I realize that she is telling me how, at the beginning of our meeting, we were communicating in a false, pseudo-adult register. I don't know yet how to say all this when I notice that the figure in the drawing has no nose. I point this out to her, and she answers that this is so that she *'won't smell unpleasant odours'*.

I can't help picking up on this and giving expression to her fear that we might avoid 'smelling' something unpleasant. She immediately tells me a heart-rending story: 'and that little girl's puppy was poisoned, and later it was hurt and broke its backbone . . . it was treated . . . but it can't have children, or else it'll die'. We had stupidly erected a defence to protect ourselves from something that might exceed the capacity of our minds to tolerate pain.

Obtuse Clarabella, the obtuseness of adults, even the obtuseness of the 'field' in the first minutes of our meeting were nothing but the defences, the 'bastion' that protected us from the feeling that she had been poisoned in her most vital and natural part, 'the puppy', and that she too was a 'broken girl', terrified that she might not be able to deliver thoughts and emotions lest she die (from pain). Coming to realize all this together with Mariella makes it possible to discuss with her the need for an analytic treatment.

Working-through as a locus of asymmetry: Franco

At the beginning of the session, 9-year-old Franco does a drawing of an aeroplane, describing it as he adds details and colours it in (Figure 2.8). I wonder what that plane is trying to tell me, how I can think about it and interpret it. But aside from a purely content-based interpretation, which does not seem to help, nothing else comes to mind. I am struck by a feeling of

Figure 2.7

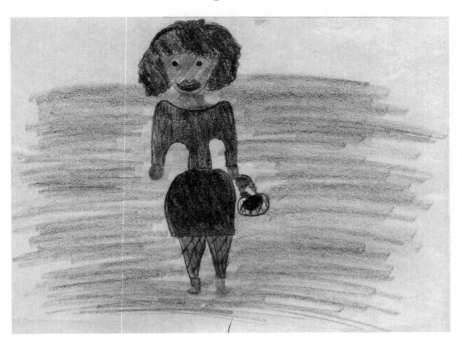

uneasiness as I look at the lines that outline the camouflage markings on the plane, and I think: 'It looks as if there are cracks in the cockpit and wings. I'd never board a plane with cracks in it like that.'

It is only at this stage that I remember that at a certain point in the preceding session I had lacked interpretive restraint, incapable as I was of 'keeping something in' that would have required more time before it could be said without having traumatic effects on Franco. I link the two facts and think Franco is telling me that, since our work is just beginning, he feels that his faith in our 'means' is cracking and that at the same time he is trying to camouflage, to hide this crisis of faith, even from himself.

I decide that all this cannot be communicated directly to Franco since it would be 'too much' for his mind to digest in its present state. I also conclude that, while continuing to follow him against the background of his narrative, in which there now appears a conflict between two opposing sides, I must manage to regain that mental and interpretive attitude which will enable me to weld together the cracks in his faith.

At the same time I notice that there is a problem of 'impulsiveness', that I had acted out by taking on Franco's projective identifications, or rather,

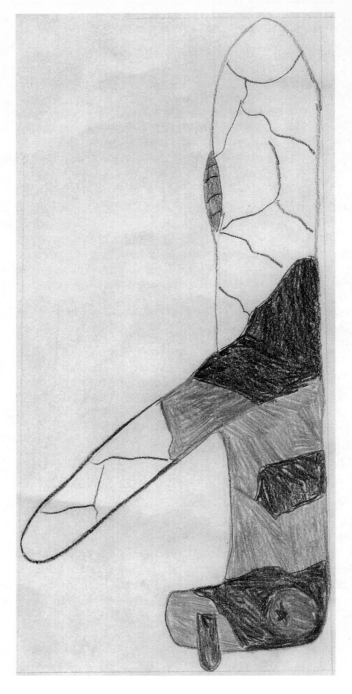

Figure 2.8

those of his incontinent parts which, in collusion with mine, had provoked the interpretive enactment. These parts were now in conflict with thought functions. In Franco's narrative text we speak of a conflict between a violent, impulsive army rashly launching an attack against a well-organized, regular army capable of 'thinking' before putting its plans into action.

The seductions of 'symbolic' interpretation: Marina

At our first meeting 10-year-old Marina does a drawing (Figure 2.9) whose contents seem to suggest an infinite number of readings: one could easily spot 'breasts', 'penises' and 'nipples', combined in such a way as to suggest geographic confusion (Meltzer 1967) of the type 'breast-bottom', 'penis-nipple', 'front-back'. But which of the various interpretive paths is the right one? While I am thinking, wondering disorientedly what tangle Marina has inside, it is Marina herself who shows the way by spontaneously associating with the drawing. She says that she doesn't know whether it reminds her more of a lollipop on a stick or of the ears and trunk of an elephant.

Marina's communication could direct our attention toward bodily phantasies, the breast/penis bipolarity. But the girl's words echo my own doubts. I am inclined to grasp the mental qualities of the communication in the here and now, that is, to pick up on the question Marina is asking herself about this stranger and about the type of relationship she will be able to have with him. Will the analyst be open and affectionate, someone with whom it will be possible to have a positive contact, or will he be violent and intrusive, someone who launches attacks with his interpretations?

The second hypothesis is clearly suggested in the scene taken from a comic book that Marina brings to a later session (Figure 2.10). This picture shows me that it is useful to stick to Marina's text in an effort to help her pose questions and formulate answers, according to the way in which I interact with her, whether lightly and gently, or heavily and obtusely. [Dialogue in the comic book frame: Dragon: 'And this is nothing! I know some interpretations that are even more interesting!' Parrot: 'Poor me!']

Drawings and the mental functioning of the couple: Marcello

Marcello, at an important moment of the analysis, seems to help me understand the two different ways of mental functioning with which I approach him. In a drawing (Figure 2.11) I am depicted in one half as sitting in front of him with a book in my hand while he is alone, going 'beep beep' with the pocket electronic game he always keeps handy. He seems to be saying that I

Figure 2.9

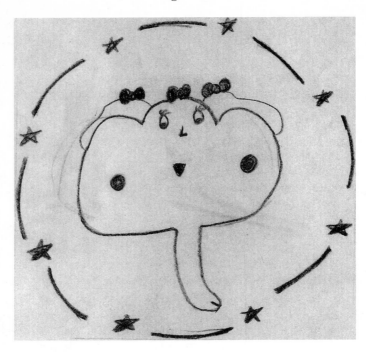

Figure 2.10

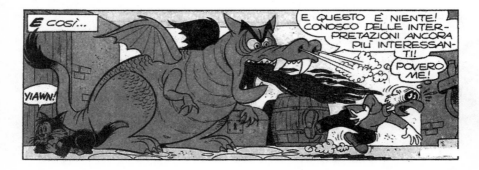

Figure 2.11

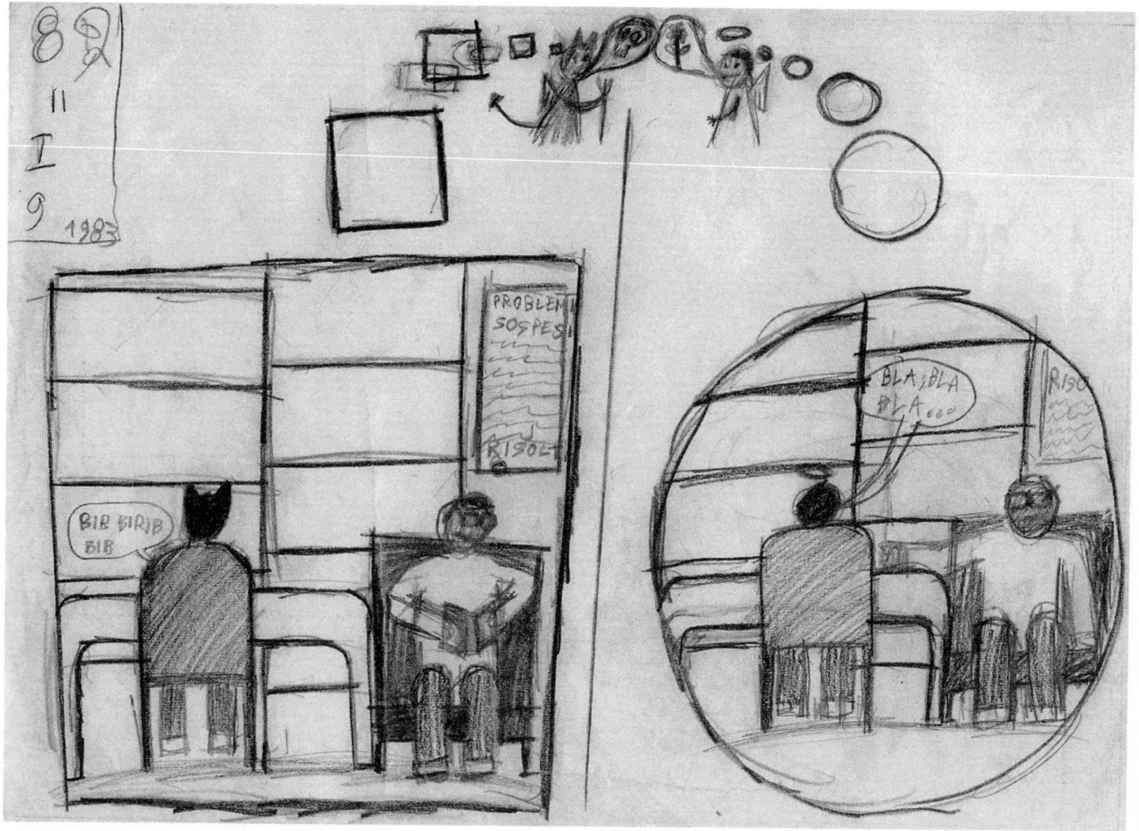

am there with my book of theories and symbols, while he goes back to being a little mechanical, electronic boy. In the other half of the picture I am holding out my hand as though it were a bridge, and he speaks to me.

There is another interesting detail. In the left half, there is a poster on the wall behind me. At the top it reads 'PROBLEMI SOSPESI' [unsolved problems]. Then there are scribbles indicating dense writing. At the bottom we read 'PROBLEMI RISOLTI = 0' [solved problems = 0], which seems to say: 'We're not making any progress this way.' In the right-hand half we find, in the middle of the poster, 'RISO', the rest of the phrase not fitting into the frame. Below there are again marks indicating a lot more writing.

This is how problems can be solved, Marcello seems to be suggesting. But there is also an emotion, no longer the 'beep beep' of the mechanical boy, but the 'riso' [laugh], that is, the expression of emotion which can be voiced only in this way, at a distance, communicated by Marcello, the boy, who feels he is being listened to and understood. What is more we find 'riso' [rice], a nutritious food which plays an important role in the long journey toward overcoming anorexia, which was one of the reasons which brought Marcello to analysis in the first place.

Of course, seen from the point of view of field dynamics the drawing calls up two oscillating modes of functioning of the couple: one angular and robotic, and the other 'round' and affectionate, in other words two ways for the minds in the field to interact. But it also contains precious information which may help the analyst and his working-through by shifting the oscillation to the right-hand side of the picture: towards a genuine process of shared emotional symbolizing, which may allow Marcello to accept emotions which, for him, have been as inaccessible as food.

Drawings and reverie: Massimo

Any approach to drawings, regardless of the interpretive code we might choose to apply, reflects a defence against rendering ourselves fully permeable to them, which is the sole prerequisite for their being reworked in dreams. Consequently, it is impossible to predict precisely how a drawing will resonate inside us, or what detail will activate our capacity for reverie.

One day Massimo draws a picture in which he depicts the entrance to the apartment building where I live: my home as he imagines it. I search for meanings and am tempted to appeal to theories and to decode symbols, but as I manage to give up remembering theories and trying to understand, Massimo continues quickly with his perfect drawing until he gets to the caption of his picture. Then he stops to ask me: 'But what do you call that thing in the corner,

AIU . . . AIU . . . AIUole [flowerbed], and he writes the word in blue★, whereas all the other words of the caption are written in black.

As soon as I understand the request for help made by Massimo the boy, who uses the picture drawn by Massimo the architect, he can begin to talk to me about his cat and about how it suffers when it is left alone at home. It is the last session of the week, and the first time that Massimo has mentioned the pain of separation.

Massimo, a boy without needs, or a boy who has always thought he could satisfy his needs by himself, is missing someone. But this communication becomes possible only after he has felt that I am tuned in and receptive to his call for help, an appeal which no theory would have enabled me to receive.

Drawings and their transformations over time: Massimo

So far I have given priority to the drawing as a dream-like frame of the relational moment, something that reveals the microtransformations in the session. This can be seen in the sequence of drawings as well as in the dialogue, both of which clearly reveal the unstable and reversible transformations of the relational moment, that in turn reflect the changing emotional structure of the analytic couple. But there is another vertex which is no less important: that of the stable and irreversible transformations considered over extended periods of time.

The following sequence of three pictures (Figures 2.12, 2.13, 2.14) reflects two years of therapy with Massimo. In these drawings, almost worthy of an engineer, human-like figures are initially quite mechanized and rigid (Figure 2.12), but gradually they begin to resemble the face of a child (Figure 2.13) who seems to be peeping out surreptitiously and unexpectedly from behind the metallic structure of a ship or a tank. Occasionally it will be the bow of a landing craft or a control panel that almost secretively takes the form of a boy seeking to emerge, to give himself structure, to gain recognition in the midst of Massimo's autistic-mechanized figures.

Then Massimo produces a picture of Pinocchio (Figure 2.14). He is still disjointed, in desperate need of his foster father, and he seems capable of expressing pain by means of the 'big spike in his heart', as Massimo puts it, as he draws a spiked paper fastener pointing towards the heart at the right of the picture.

Considered within the context of years of work, these are stable *and irreversible* transformations which may be viewed not only in terms of the

---

★ Translator's note: AIU, the letters written in blue, are the first three of the Italian word AIUTO = help.

Figure 2.12

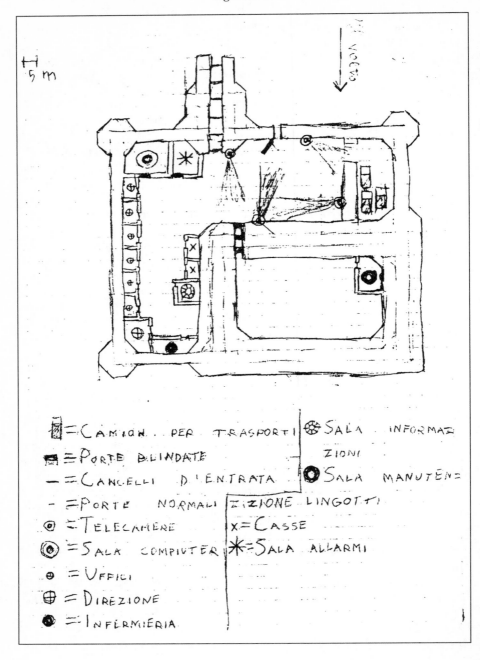

Figure 2.13

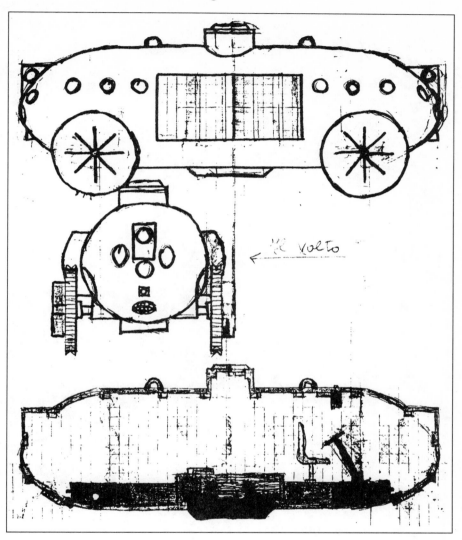

changes taking place in Massimo's internal world and in his mode of functioning, but also as an expression of the changes in the interaction of the patient's and the analyst's minds in the session. We are moving from a more mechanized, controlled approach towards greater spontaneity, until we are finally able to achieve and share full contact with the pain and suffering which leads to integration and change.

Figure 2.14

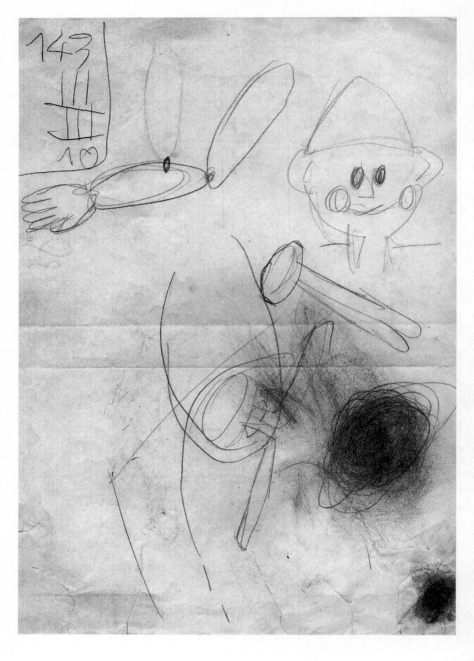

Drawing as emergency

I would now like to describe other situations, besides the normal one in which a child does a drawing in the consulting room or brings one from home. These are situations in which drawings have nonetheless contributed, though in different ways, to the analysis of a patient.

A drawing done by the analyst during the session: Renato

The first time I see Renato he reminds me of a bison-calf, and this is what he turns out to be, as he contains himself in almost muscular fashion (Bick 1968) with the hyperactivity he uses to protect himself from catastrophic total dissolution.

There is nothing I am able to say that has any effect on his running, no matter at what level I try to communicate. On the contrary, my speaking seems to goad him, as though my words were bullets. In response he picks up some wooden blocks and throws them at me, almost hitting and hurting me.

I try to tell him I feel like a cowboy surrounded by attacking Indians, but nothing will stop him. The perimeter of his running track extends to the waiting room and he continues to run around with his head lowered. I'm beginning to think that it would take a fence to keep him in and I am actually tempted to make one, at least within the confines of the room. Instead, I am still there in my chair, drawing a fence on one of the sheets of paper I had prepared for him. He stops, more curious than interested.

He picks up a coloured pencil and, making big marks outside the boundary of the fence, says: 'And I'm going to break it, I'm going to break it.' Then he draws a red funnel. I say it looks like a whirlwind, or a tornado, or maybe Red Cloud, who can break through any fence.

Still standing, he says: 'Draw more fences!' I obey, wondering if I'm acting out, but at the same time trying desperately to think. He continues to break the fences with the same coloured turbine. I say it looks as if there is no dam that could hold him back.

I keep making fences and inside one fenced area I draw something like a table. He takes a felt-tipped pen to the wall and on a tile draws 'an Indian teepee'. I say: 'A place for Red Cloud.'

On my sheet he draws a teepee, an Indian child and a whirlwind. In the meantime I am thinking about how, while running round, he has not only overturned the toy box but also knocked over chairs, side tables and so forth. It looks like a battlefield. I remember how his mother told me that when Renato has one of his frequent uncontrolled fits in which he tries to break everything in sight the only thing that stops him is cartoons.

He comes closer and, instead of using the wall tiles as a drawing pad, this time he uses the tabletop and draws an Indian boy picking up everything that has fallen out of a basket 'With the help of his friend the crab who has arms that pinch without hurting.' He continues drawing, 'But as the two friends are working somebody shoots at them . . . then another cyclone strikes.'

The session continues. But now we have these 'characters' we have created together in our animated cartoon, characters that will help us give a name to and turn into story what happens in the room and between our two minds. This is the necessary precondition for the recognition, narration and transformation of emotions and feelings, which is what Lussana meant (1991) when speaking of the evolution from Kleinian to Bionian interpretation.

One could debate whether my drawing was an acting out, a question dealt with by Schlesinger (1989). I would observe, however, that denying oneself a certain freedom in emergency situations would mean sacrificing to formalistic rigour what can in fact be communicated and transformed, albeit with exceptional and apparently improper means. For, basically, my drawings reveal three things: the incapacity to think enough, a need to discharge (like Renato's physical running) and the need for a dam, a boundary, which, once erected, would allow the transformations and shared thought processes to take place.

Needless to say, I considered all the characters of the session to be functions and holograms of the couple and of the emotional exchanges between the two of us. They were a point of departure for the narration of emotions and feelings which turned from an incontinent mode toward a mode in which thought and verbal communication become possible. As proto-characters are born, they bear witness to what I have called 'functional aggregates', to which I will return at the end of this chapter and in the chapter on dialogue.

Dreaming up a drawing: Carlo's black spot

Carlo is a 7-year-old boy who is trying to contain, to find a place for, and to distinguish feelings which previously had been violently evacuated. In the session he has a furious fit of jealousy, partly connected with the traces left by another boy from the previous hour.

Before his outburst of jealousy Carlo had made a drawing for me. It had struck me because it showed the boy's new ability to keep the colours (feelings?) inside the lines. At the same time, however, I was unsettled by a black spot which I didn't know what to make of, dark parts, destructive parts?

Then Carlo has his fit of jealousy. Because I don't know how to stop him as he screams and throws everything on the floor, I interpret this furious, angry jealousy, quite actively but ineffectively, about someone else having entered the room. Once the crisis has passed, Carlo says: 'That's not what you're supposed to say to me when I feel bad. I just get angrier. You should give me something that belongs to you, so that I understand I'm not alone and you're not cross with me. That way I smile and I calm down.'

I'm struck by what he says, and wonder what he is asking of me and why he tells me that such direct interpretations are ineffective, even harmful. I think about what I can do with him.

That night I have a dream. In the children's consulting room I see something black walking, almost crawling, on the wall. I don't understand what it is and I move toward it. It is a 'black spot' that seems to be walking; no, it's a cockroach, getting bigger and bigger. I don't know what to do, and it seems to me that I don't have the right equipment. Cautiously I pick up a stick and confront it. I hit it as hard as I can, harder and harder, more and more uselessly. The cockroach just gets angrier and moans.

When I wake up I realize that the dream has helped me understand how threatened I felt by the black spot, a hole in understanding, perhaps an unthinkable zone in Carlo's mind, but at the same time a dark, unthought zone in our relationship; and I realize how I was protecting myself from that zone by attacking him with evacuative, defensive pseudo-interpretations.

Perhaps the right approach is not to interpret anger and jealousy so actively, but rather to reflect on Carlo's words, to consider the path that he himself suggests when he says 'give me something that belongs to you, so that I can understand . . . that you're not cross with me'. Perhaps I should be able to offer him the capacity of my analyst's mind to transform emotions and thoughts in the session, setting aside rigid and preconstituted schemes, which are a source of certainty for me but of desperation for my patient. So I have to wait for our two minds to produce something together, as Carlo will confirm in a later dream: in a room, there appears 'something horrible with hair sprouting on its body and head which, if somebody stays close to it and helps it, will grow and take shape'. In another dream we find 'a little black boy who goes into the forest to meet the animals that live there'.

Interpretations, then, can sometimes serve as a defence against the expansion of the mind, to allow us to avoid recognizing our own more animal, primitive parts, our 'monsters', our rejected parts (Neri *et al.* 1989). Such parts may emerge precisely in the meeting and in the exchange of projective identifications with the patient, as a precondition for the emotional field to take shape and for affects to become communicable.

Several months later, Carlo draws a picture (using the same colours) in which there appears a 7-year-old boy who, like a Russian doll, contains another small boy of a year and a half who is about to have a birthday and who is growing where the black spot was. Now, instead of the black spot, there is a child part that it had not been possible to think about before, whose needs had not been recognizable, and which gradually assumes a structure and acquires a 'body', where once there was the black spot. So it was not jealousy or destructiveness but a 'lump' of a child's needs that had to be 'shaped' and subsequently recognized.

Drawing a dream: Salvino's keys

Salvino, 12 years old, is in an advanced stage of analysis, and we have still not managed to set a date for the end of our work (in part due to particular facts in the patient's life). When Salvino is worried that I might not understand his need to end the analysis, he has a dream in which there is a door which may now be opened thanks to some keys whose 'heads are changed, although the bodies are the same'.

Concerned that he will not be able to express the meaning of his dream, Salvino brings in some sheets of paper on which he has tried to draw 'keys with their heads changed but with the same body', where 'head' means the part of the key with the notches and 'body' the part held in the hand. It was a different internal composition, then, a different notching that allowed him to open the door to mourning and to the end of the analysis. The picture satisfied the need to show me concretely the changes in internal composition and structure which Salvino feared I could not yet see clearly.

A drawing of the countertransference outside the session

A therapist who has for some time been under my supervision for the psychotherapy of a very small boy brings me, during the boy's absence, the session report of an 8-year-old girl. The therapist, whom I have observed to be very attentive to problems of the setting, tells me, as if it were not particularly important, that for the last two years she has begun sessions by giving the girl four sweets while keeping the same number for herself. Then she gives two of her own to the girl and eats the other two. The girl, for her part, eats four and keeps two for after the session.

I am amazed by this account but say nothing. I'm reminded of a lion tamer in a circus who, before entering the ring, is so afraid of the beasts that he gives them sedatives, reserving a dose for himself which he then cuts in half considering it more urgent to calm down the animals.

The session goes on with pictures, drawn by the girl, of a man and a woman. In the course of the hour the girl makes numerous holes in the paper with the sharp pencil points. The therapist interprets something concerning the difference between the sexes and castration anxieties connected with the broken pencil points. (I, on the other hand, think of the dagger stabs inflicted by Brutus, or rather by a brute.) It is clear that the therapist is not thinking and that she is paralysed with terror. I might say that she is incapable of doing her job, but this is not the case as I have seen her work competently in various and difficult situations. If I consider the child's material, it is obvious that she feels homicidal rage towards the therapist (mother and father?). But if I consider the analytic couple, I can understand more: there is a paralysis of thought, a fear that leads the therapist to administer sedative sweets and a terror that makes her say totally senseless things in the face of the girl's fury, a fury that grows as the therapist's defences increase.

Almost by chance, the therapist shows me a drawing (Figure 2.15) she made herself after this session. There is a black, savage girl with a lance and her head full of red feathers (a head in flames?). She is standing in front of a hut made of leaves with two windows at the sides and a door in the middle. The therapist remarks: 'It looks like the house of one of the three little pigs . . . the straw hut.'

Figure 2.15

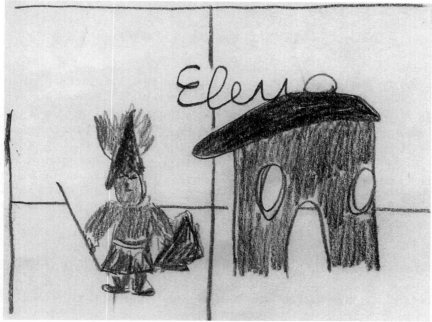

Here, then, is the interpretive key that the psychotherapist herself provides. There is a savage little cannibal, violent and primitive, and the therapist, whose shocked face seems to recur in the hut with its wide-open window eyes and open door mouth. The therapist is terrified that she will not be able to take in and contain the little savage, afraid of being overcome and disorganized as a container.

Another observation might be added. Neither the therapist's acting out (the sweets) nor the interpretive acting out (the defensive interpretations) are really important here. What counts is the incapacity to think it necessary to metabolize these facts.

In this connection, I cannot help recalling a story told to me by a psychotic patient – I don't remember whether taken from his family history or from a film – about a ferocious boxer whose opponents used to send him call girls to wear him out so that he would be more manageable in the ring. Needless to say, I too used clever means to calm down my patient and then landed my interpretive punches only when I felt the situation was under my control. My patient's suggestion, however, helped me work through just how afraid I was of him.

This shows clearly how the analyst's defences structure and modify the field. Consequently, the suffering of countertransference and self-analysis becomes a necessary tune-up for an instrument continually subjected to stress. The characters of the sessions, drawings and dreams constantly provide occasions and tools for this sort of work.

Drawings in the analysis of adults

There is a classic precedent for this in Milner's splendid analysis of Susan (1969). Fachinelli (1983), too, has published some graphic material furnished by a patient in the course of analysis. But as this is not common, it may be useful to present another example of how an adult patient's drawing (Figure 2.16) reveals my untimely tendency to dig for meanings before emotions and affects have gained free passage. The two frames of the drawing show an evident change in facial expression, from radiant joy to sad disappointment. This suggests that I provided an answer that reflected intellectual rumination rather than a willingness to share with the patient his 'amazed wonder' at all the comets which, to paraphrase Di Chiara's (1990) suggestive metaphor, may appear in the consulting room.

Words as 'drawing' in the relationship, during analysis of adults

As I feel it is important to stress how languages are open to transformation as well as to play down the differences between the analysis of children and

Figure 2.16

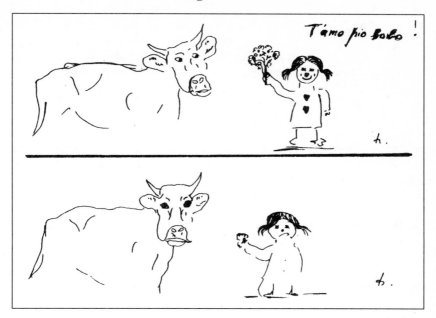

adults, I would like to show by means of a brief clinical illustration how the 'words' uttered in the consulting room are similar to drawings within the relationship.

It was Tiziana who induced me to think clearly about the verbal text of a session much as I would think about a picture drawn with words. This occurred in a period in which I was particularly attentive to the question of communication, understood as communication in the transference and therefore constantly requiring explicit formulation.

Since adolescence Tiziana has been 'going steady' with a promising young student at a Fine Arts Academy and she has a very intense relationship with him. In the analysis, her 'artist' boyfriend takes on two forms: at times he is the analyst himself in his interpretive frescoes, in the texture and composition of his utterances; at other times, he is a part of the patient that oscillates between two organizational modalities, one narcissistic-destructive, the other creative.

The narcissistic mode is the 'boyfriend that destroys his pictures' (when the patient does not bring any dreams) and the creative one is 'the boyfriend that paints and keeps his pictures' (the patient brings dreams). But this reflects in turn two interpretive modes of the analyst (in an infinite game of self-reflecting mirrors), the narcissistic analyst (Brenman, 1977) who destroys the 'pictures', if only because he stimulates envy and competitiveness in the patient, and the creative analyst, a result of the link ($♀$ $♂$) with the patient.

For some time Tiziana is in touch with the emotional quality and tonality in her boyfriend's paintings, in my interpretations and in her internal world. 'My boyfriend paints according to the way colours go together', she says. So the affective tonality of my interpretations is perceived as a whole, and her attention, at first, is directed towards how her own sensations take shape, organize and distinguish themselves almost chromatically. Only later will her boyfriend 'adopt a figurative technique'.

At this point it will be possible for Tiziana to grasp the *descriptive contents* of my interpretations and the figurative elements of her own emotions. In this way I become aware of the qualities of my verbal painting, of the shading of tones, of certain characteristics of my colours, and I 'learn to paint' from the patient who teaches me to make paintings which correspond increasingly to what she feels and experiences in the session.

But the patient also 'learns to paint' from me, and I teach her how to proceed from a purely chromatic depiction of sensations to a figurative technique, which entails the recognition and description of her own feelings and emotions. Two of Tiziana's dreams bear witness to this development. In the first there appears a Renaissance woman with red hair (and a plait) with whom Tiziana associates the French actress Fanny Ardant. In the second I am giving a swallow some tufts of cotton to make a nest with. Thus the dream narrates the successful process of creating a 'place' which can hold her ardent thoughts and feelings. That was a problem which had occupied us ever since she brought in a 'pastel' her boyfriend had made depicting a wounded girl with a slash, or rather a white blade, in her abdomen which indicated the lack of a uterus: a uterus for children, a mental place for feelings and passions.

The meagre meal ['pasto'] ('pastels' were to dominate the boyfriend's work for some time) consists of cotton tufts which will serve to build Tiziana's ability to think and experience emotions autonomously. After years of exhausting evacuative 'chocolate cakes', we will find her busy mixing, sifting, trying out new ingredients and new ways of putting them together in her affective kitchen: until finally she produces 'crêpes', through which, amidst anger ('Crepa!' [Go to hell!]) and pain ('Crepo!' [I'm dying!]), she will develop the ability to create something new, the fruit of working and thinking.

As we see, if the analyst's attention is directed to the here and now of the relationship, the interpretation is conditioned by the patient's response as regards 'speed-distance' (Meltzer, 1976), but it remains a direct and explicit interpretation of the relationship.

Patients themselves have suggested that this *hic et nunc* approach to listening is 'too tight'. It may create too much closeness, that could result from phantasies of undifferentiation. It may also stifle the creative liberty of the couple at work and the freedom of the patient's mind to generate 'thoughts' which are not subject to the continual denial that often arises from the unavoidable shifting of plane and meaning brought about by strong, unambiguous interpretations.

Perhaps, then, interpretations can be considered in a different way, a way that brings together two different approaches: on the one hand, Bion's conceptions of 'unsaturatedness' and of the time required to communicate an intuition; on the other, the Barangers' emphasis on the 'couple'. We should here remember that the Barangers always refer to the 'unconscious phantasy of the couple', which needs the analyst's 'second look' in order to be mobilized. This is rather different from other approaches which refer to more phenomenological aspects of the patient–analyst couple. The Barangers emphasize that the analytic situation consists of a bi-personal field which is structured, in equal measure, by both analyst and patient, although the former is responsible for the modulation of the events of the field. It is the bringing together of these two points of view that makes the perspective presented in the following section possible.

Word drawings in the field

The entire dialogue of the session, then, seems to resemble increasingly a drawing with rather peculiar characteristics, its components constantly in motion as in a living picture.

The setting provides the frame, and the emotions of the couple the canvas and colours, which are in turn brought together and organized by the words. Gradually the words themselves acquire a form and a structure: most commonly as characters, tales, stories, which may be about animals, plants, minerals and so on. But these figurations, which vary with the changes in the emotional and relational set-up of the couple, are the only way the two minds have of telling each other what is happening between them, especially through the exchange of projective identifications.

It is fascinating, from this point of view, to observe how a 'character' enters the session, moves about, changes and exits, only to be replaced by, or combined with, another 'character' (of an anecdote, a memory, a story, a dream), but always contributing form and colour to what is happening in the mental functioning of the couple at a particular moment.

Different models interact in different ways according to the 'living pictures' of the sessions. Even those with greater claim to neutrality enter into the construction of the field, since interpretations often serve as defences of the analyst's mind against the mental pain which it cannot assimilate and transform.

It follows from this approach that the analyst must accept full awareness of and responsibility for the role that her mental life plays in structuring, together with the patient, the emotional, affective and linguistic field. She is also responsible for bringing to life, from among the many possible stories, the unique and unrepeatable story which emerges from the analytic encounter, with all its creative wealth and specific mutilations. And if this is true for the entire course of the analysis, it is equally true for each of its sub-units, whether it be a week or an hour.

This model forces us to ask: 'What have I got to do with what is taking shape in the field?' But the question does not imply mere Freudian repetition compulsion nor the Kleinian patient's projected phantasies. Rather, it is a signal from the patient, though from a vertex for the moment unknown to us, about what is happening in the session.

At the same time we must be aware that the flow of influences is reciprocal: that is, not only does the analyst influence the patient, but the patient also influences the analyst in a circular movement not only of the 'analytic dialogue', as Nissim Momigliano would put it (1984), but also and above all in the continual and reciprocal exchange of projective identifications. From this perspective our 'best colleague', the patient (Bion 1980), serves as a coxswain who gives us a running account of what is happening from a different point of view. I think it would be meaningless to utilize this interpretive level by making it explicit, as Langs seems to suggest (1975, 1978). The captain, I feel, should only make use of these signals to keep the ship on course; the course, that is, which allows the psychotic parts of the personality to achieve those 'realizations' they have never had before.

If, after a session which the analyst has considered particularly intense, the young patient says that her sister ate too much risotto too quickly and then got congested and lost her senses, this is a signal for the analyst that an exces-sively intense and condensed emotional charge (risotto: 'riso' [rice]/food; 'riso' [laugh]/emotion) for the sister 'function' causes a loss of sense (faint-ing/losing connections), and that the interpretive and relational register must be decreased in order to avoid 'loss of meaning'.

Another little girl dreams of poisonous snakes approaching her while her mother tells her not to worry, and of her father putting her behind the steer-ing wheel of a fast car. Then she dreams of meeting the analyst in the street. She almost runs into her and throws her own daughter at her, while at the same time separating the patient's hand from her mother's. In this case the analyst can hardly help asking what makes the snakes move and where are the father who has the girl drive a car that goes too fast and the mother who does not perceive danger. She will also think that the daughter thrown at the girl was a 'correct' interpretation, but thought out by herself alone and simply tossed at the patient. This was the case, for example, when I inter-preted 'the brother who has it in for southern Italians' as an aggressive part of the patient who was angry with the analyst. But it was not yet time to say so. There was in the field a little girl who still needed her mother to hold back this 'dangerous brother'.

It is clear that this intratextual, or rather subtextual, level cannot be interpreted for the patient. Indeed, the entire session may be seen as a countertransference dream which will help the analyst regulate her mental and interpretive asset so that she can find the specific functions which the patient needs, for example 'a mother who keeps her close', who understands the danger of hurrying and of the sudden, and perhaps inappropriate, bringing together of the split-off parts of the personality – which, after all, need not always be those of the patient.[1]

The concept of dependence is here turned upside down. It is no longer the patient who must be dependent, accepting the analyst's food/child interpretations as the patient's neurotic parts basically do, but rather the analyst who must be able to depend on the patient's emotional needs. If a patient says 'my father is away at work too long, spends too much time at the hospital and too little time at home with the family, and he never holds our hands or puts us on his lap', we are not dealing with erotization. Rather, we are dealing with a request for the analyst to change his mental functioning, to interpret and work less (explicitly), to be manifestly receptive to the patient's needs, respecting his text and thereby functioning as a father who is affectionate and keeps you close, rather than one who is always away at work.

In the *living pictures* that the couple create in the session there are numerous interferences and disturbances, often generated by the analyst himself who, ultimately, functions (and must function) as the capacious recipient of the patient's projective identifications. The analyst, as such, becomes the vehicle for the entrance of that mental functioning which the patient will call 'X' or will introduce through the character 'Z'.

It is not so much the interpretation that shakes the field as the reception of the patient's signal concerning what is happening that allows a gradual modification of the interventions and thereby the transformation of the 'characters' of the session as an expression of the emotional climate of the couple at work (Ferro 1991, 1994). But all this will become clearer in Chapter 4, which deals with dialogue.

A few reflections

I will leave the clinical sequences I have presented without further comment as I feel that the underlying model can be easily inferred from the situations described. I will limit myself to a brief mention of the possibility of identifying, also through drawings in progress , 'functional aggregates' (as in the example of the bison-calf, the aeroplane, or the transformations of the Pinocchio Robot). There is always a vertex from which the drawing can be seen as a 'functional aggregate'. It is on this point that I would like to add a few observations.

The exchange between analyst and patient is broader than the mere verbal exchange, and alongside words there are other modes of communication, especially through reciprocal projective identifications. If that is true, it is consequently not always immediately possible to assign split-off parts and ways of functioning to one of the members of the pair and to determine how they condition the events of the session. Rosenfeld (1987) underlines how the patient is able to dream the split-off parts of the analyst's mind and how these parts can interfere with her mental and interpretive organization.

The dreams we have at night, whether we remember them or not, are for both Bion and Meltzer a sort of sample of an ongoing process which unfolds when we are asleep as well as when we are awake. In the same way there is a dream-like functioning of the two minds in the session which dream one another in the reciprocal flow of stimuli and projective identifications. In our waking state we can find the derivatives of this 'dream' as they emerge in phantasies, images, associations, narrations and, in certain particular situations, dream-like snapshots of the waking state, which are real images of the dream projected outwards (see Chapter 4).

Seen from this perspective the characters, the narrations, the memories and the drawings, for example, can be rethought as 'syntheses of functioning' of the analytic couple at a particular moment, which continually change and transform according to the way they interact and to the quality of this interaction.

Bezoari and I coined the term 'functional aggregate' to define, within an almost transitional area, the composition of a 'character'[2] which cannot always be easily attributed to one or other actor/author on the analytic stage. Are we dealing with a part of you, a part of me, a projected part of you, a projected part of you and assumed by me, or assumed by me with the addition of something of my own? And how much of my own? (Also in the inversions of flow: parts of me projected and received by you, and how much of your own? And so on ad infinitum.) In other words, we are talking about the set of problems posed by the *strong, relational conception* of projective identifications and of role assumption, such as that which emerge in the works mentioned in this connection in Chapter 7.

All these are varying forms and attributions which must often remain indeterminate for some time before we can explicitly define their relational status. It is worth stressing that what really counts is not the explicit definition of the status but how these 'forms' undergo gradual transformation in the game of mental interactions.

We are used to thinking in terms of split-off parts. We have long misused such clumsy interpretations as 'It is a part of you that . . .', as if it were possible for the analyst to be nothing more than a mirror, as if she did not participate in structuring the field she contributes to defining. We have played down the problems concerning how to regard the characters brought to the session, whether they are figures from external reality, or parts of the internal world, or aspects of the patient projected into characters of the real world. The problem can be nullified if the character, the drawing, or even the whole of the patient's communication is viewed from a vertex which makes us focus exclusively on characters (or narrations) which are pertinent to the session and which constitute the variable function and outcome of the functioning of the couple. After all, the functional aggregate is none other than the opposite of the Barangers' concept of the bastion: it is a variable communication flow as opposed to a static, solidified precipitate of reciprocal projective identifications which crystallizes the situation (as in the impasse or role assumption) and determines a fixed position (Gear *et al.* 1976).

Of course, all this is true for drawings, games and dialogues, where it will be even easier to show the approach at work.

3

Play

Introduction

Before talking about play, I would like to make a few observations on fairy tales, as I feel that play is very much like a personal fairy tale which children make up as they go along.

Play originates in the early relationship of a caring mother with her child. Their games often consist in making faces and noises, and such activities are highly communicative (Stern 1977, 1985). This communication is accompanied by the exchange of projective identifications transmitting emotional and affective states. The child's projections are then received, metabolized and transformed by the mother's reverie (Bion, 1962, 1967b; Bordi, 1980). These primary relationships constitute the soil that gives rise to both fairy tales and play.

That the child's inner world is populated by terrifying contents is confirmed by her fascination for fairy tales. Many of these are cruel, like 'Little Red Riding Hood', 'Thumbellina' and 'Blue Beard'. Others are peopled with witches and stepmothers, and their characters are moulded by revenge, envy and jealousy.

The importance of fairy tales for the mental development of a child rests, I believe, on two essential factors. First of all, they are *unsaturated*, so each child can fill in a fairy tale with different meanings, depending on his or her stage of growth or emotional state. Second, there is the emotional plot that child and storyteller create. What has the potential to transform the child's deepest phantasies is 'living' and activated not so much by the narrated text as by the affective and emotional fabric which is woven by child and narrator together (Ferro 1985c).

Children live in a state of constant dependency. They have urgent needs and strong emotions. They are always afraid that their needs will remain unsatisfied and they are afraid of the needs they project outward. A striking illustration of this is described by Isaacs (1948), drawing on an observation reported by Jones. A small child looks at his mother's breast as she is feeding his little brother and says: 'That's what you used to bite me with.'

Fairy tales provide children with representations of their own most terrible and hidden fears and depict their own expectations, both ideal and idealized. Children often like to listen to these stories in the evening before they go to sleep. The setting of many fairy tales, moreover, is a dark wood, which recreates the darkness of the bedroom and the blackness of sleep. The encounters in the stories, many of which are frightening, are meetings with the phantasies and dreams which work on the day's events and produce new and unforeseen connections.

Fairy tales are also set in worlds distant both in time and space ('once upon a time') and often in mythical places (Sicilian tales, for instance, often refer to the 'Little Princedom of Portugal'). This remoteness allows a child to live with those fears that he could never admit stem from encounters with the people he holds dearest. A child cannot bear to think, for example, that the witch and the ogre are also ways in which he sees the mother and father he needs so much, or that they are parts of his own self, or feelings which take shape in his most intimate relationships. Infanticides, matricides and devourings, all events which dominate the phantasy world of children and adults, are split and sent off to a separate foreign land. Once an 8-year-old boy, in analysis, invented another world ('the world of points of view') to contain the phantasies and emotions which he could not tolerate living with in his own world.

The fairy tale also allows the child to identify with the characters and to experience the tale from within. This permits her to metabolize her most terrible feelings by entrusting them to and receiving them back from the story. The fairy tale can perform the function of the mother who makes herself permeable to the child's fears and returns them to her in less terrifying form. Thumbellina gets lost in the wood, just as every child does in her emotions, but the fairy tale tells her that there is a *remedy*. This seems to me to be the key factor, together with the stories' capacity to *contain*: children are in fact afraid that their feelings, fears, emotions and instincts are uncontainable, and that there is a risk of being overwhelmed by them. Fairy tales show that a solution can be found even to situations perceived as catastrophic and irreparable.

Furthermore, through fairy tales the child discovers that her fears can be *shared*. The child learns that others have had the same experiences before her, for many of her own fears are there in the story. The fairy tale offers protection like a wise old man who has been through it all, who can understand the child, make her feel understood and above all give a name,[1] a plot and a meaning to the anxieties which she feels mysteriously pervade her. One wonders whether it might not be because of this 'ancient wisdom' that fairy tales are often transmitted by grandparents.

In *The Uses of Enchantment* Bruno Bettelheim (1975) proposes a reading of the best known fairy tales, from a psychoanalytical point of view. He chooses those which he thinks best represent the anxieties and fears of children. In my view, however, fairy tales do not in themselves completely represent the whole of children's fears and anxieties nor provide symbols for them, or at least not as completely as Bettelheim often suggests. Nor do I believe that they are as saturated with meaning as he seems to think. I believe rather that they serve as containers, recipients of various shapes and sizes, which can be filled by individual children according to their emotional needs. Fairy tales offer a sort of hypothesis of symbolization which can be used in different ways by each child. They were in fact transmitted orally before being collected and transcribed.

This is exactly what happens with what are often interpreted as symbols in dreams. Taken individually their meanings are so general that they allow no development. What generates meaning, however, is the way in which the elements come together, the bonds between the symbols, and their connections with the emotions of the teller of the dream and those of the listener. (Meltzer 1981a).

In the fairy tale, then, we can find an internal plot which is far less saturated than Bettelheim suggests. 'Little Red Riding Hood', for example, lends itself to diverging interpretations. But in considering the fairy tale/symbol interrelationship, only in its encounter with a particular child at a particular moment, and then with another child at another moment, will the numerous meanings take shape. These meanings vary according to the individual child's emotional needs in each moment of encounter with a particular narrator.

The desire to listen to the same story over and over again may reflect the persistence of a basic emotional state which leads the child to choose a particular fairy tale. On the other hand, it may also show that the child is constantly going over and reworking his own phantasies. If this is true, then the fairy tale is never truly the same: at each hearing it is perceived differently.

Similar considerations are also valid for play, whether in the consulting room or in general. Here, too, the *unsaturated* nature of play and toys (and interpretations!) is central. This aspect of play makes it possible for the child to avoid falling victim to the constraints of a game which are preconditioned by the game itself. Moreover, of fundamental importance is the *presence of an 'other'*. In other words, there must be someone to play with. Toys are like the pre-text of a narration which will unfold in the course of a shared game, a game which can be viewed as a 'cognitive, semiotic experiment' (Bertolini *et al.* 1978). A toy may by itself help the child to represent his conflicts and try to find solutions for them by himself, but it is only through the mental presence of another person playing with him (just as the fairy tale needs a narrator!) that play realizes its full potential to transform anxieties. It is the reception of the mental and emotional states present during play that permits the deepest transformations.

Every child faces the problem of passing progressively through each region of his mind (though he ought to be accompanied on this journey)[2] so that he can subsequently integrate them. Marco, whose parents could not always find sufficient mental space for him, had invented a compulsive game in which he would become robot-like and run all over the house shrieking and yelling until he hypnotized himself and fell on the floor with one hand quivering. This was the only way for him to 'self-contain' the immense anxieties which stemmed from his vision of the grown-up world as an impervious world of buses, each one following its own route without regard for the others. The game gradually came under control again as Marco's parents managed to find mental space for their son.

The introjection of a mother who knows how to tell fairy tales, or how to participate in her child's play, helps the child both to 'play by himself' (i.e. to narrate to himself what is going on inside him, distance himself from these events and find solutions) and to 'play' with other children. Moreover, this process becomes creative if there is an 'agency' constantly available to receive the anxieties that may surface in the course of play. An example of this is given by Winnicott (1965), who describes a child playing by himself *in the presence* of his mother.

As regards the analytic relationship, it is the analyst who becomes 'the setting of possible fairy tales and play'. He lends himself to all the emotional roles required by the field, roles which can subsequently be thought about again and verbalized, once they have been transformed in the analyst's working-through.

Play and psychoanalysis

Play, then, can be considered as an instrument which children use to dramatize, represent, communicate, and discharge their unconscious phantasies. It also permits children to work through and transform the anxiety and distress linked to these phantasies,[3] as well as to experience 'anticipated identifications' (Alvarez 1988).

Here is a brief explanation of how this formulation was arrived at, with reference to the work of Freud and Klein, followed by a few illustrative case studies. From the analysis of adults (if we leave aside the case of Hans who was analysed via his father) Freud drew certain inferences concerning the psychological life of children. He studied the behaviour of his own children and advised his pupils to do the same. But it was Melanie Klein who first observed children in analysis. This was not a simple task. Initially she was heavily criticized both for the pedagogical prejudices that characterized child therapy at the time (Hug–Hellmuth 1921) and for the scandal that reports of her work caused within the Psychoanalytic Society of Berlin.

Klein began by describing what she observed without really being aware of the conceptual implications that working with children might have (Segal 1979). But by 'listening' to children, as we pointed out in Chapter 1, she soon came to realize how important the 'spaces' inside their bodies are to them. However, this discovery was not widely recognized at the time, because her use of language was considered more poetic than descriptive (Meltzer 1979).

Klein believed that the observation of play provided the key to an understanding of the world of children. Play, for Klein, constitutes the child's *true work*. Play represents even the most primitive phantasies of the child and allows her to master her anxiety and work through her conflicts.

Freud had drawn attention to the play and phantasies of children on more than one occasion. He had pointed out how Hans, for example, had stuck a penknife into a hole in a doll's body and then ripped its legs open to let the knife out. With this game the child was re-enacting the phantasy of something that penetrates, and something that comes out of his mother. Not by chance was this game observed in a period when Hans was dealing with the problems of conception, his own birth and that of his little sister Hanna.

In another passage Freud gave a detailed description of the famous reel game. Here his 18-month-old grandson threw a cotton reel attached to a string out of his crib and made it disappear, saying 'fort' [away]. Then he pulled the string, made it reappear, and said happily 'da' [here]. The child played this game while his mother was away, suggesting that by controlling the appearance and disappearance of the reel he was able to control the appearance and disappearance of his mother and the attendant anxiety. Freud stressed that it was important for children to make the transition from the passivity of experiencing to the activity of playing, and that play expressed the child's desire to be a grown-up and to do the same things that grown-ups do.

Klein's innovation was to observe the child at play, exclusively from a psychoanalytic vertex and in an analytic situation. In this way every aspect of the child's behaviour and activity can help us understand what is going on in the child's mind.

The analysis of Fritz (her son Erich), a boy of 5, was conducted in his own home with his own toys. The same happened with Rita, 2 years and 2 months old (chronological age). Then Klein decided that, in order to overcome the difficulties that might arise from the proximity of the child's parents, the therapy should be carried out on the analyst's premises. She provided toys which would allow the child to express his unconscious phantasies without being influenced by the toys themselves. The toys were small and unobtrusive, so as to facilitate the best possible representation of the child's internal world and to allow the child's most primitive images to emerge and be processed.

Certain features of Klein's observational techniques are worthy of special attention. In 'The Psychological Principles of Early Analysis' (1926b) and 'On Observing the Behaviour of Young Infants' (1952b) she sets out what amounts to a manifesto of her method of observation. The main points are these:

1 To discover underlying phantasies, it is necessary to determine the connections between observed facts, emphasizing the reciprocity of each element without giving priority to any one in particular, no matter how full of symbolic meaning it might be.

2 It is necessary to consider the 'medley of factors which so often seems confused and meaningless', the 'material' that children produce, the 'manner' in which they play, the reason why they change from one to another, the 'means' they choose for their representations as a 'whole, consistent and full of meaning', which, if interpreted just like dreams, will reveal underlying phantasies and thoughts.

I will give only a few examples from the enormous amount of work Klein did with children (the cases of Fritz, Rita, Erna, Trude, Richard, etc.), underlining the theoretical enrichment, or rather revolution, which this work brought about, both in psychoanalytic theory and in our knowledge of the deepest aspects of emotional and mental life. Following Segal (1979), some of Klein's major contributions can be summarized as follows.

1 *The belief in the importance of children's aggressiveness and its links with persecutory feelings*. In line with Freud's later writings, Klein developed this conviction from observing the child's behaviour towards a toy he has damaged. If it represents a sibling or a parent, the toy is rejected. This aversion for the object derives from the fear of being persecuted. The person who is attacked, represented by the toy, is feared as vindictive and dangerous. If the child looks for the damaged toy in the toy box one day, this will mean that his persecutory anxieties have diminished, reflecting a change in his relationship with the person represented by the toy. Another example (Klein 1927b) is that of Gerald, for whom one of the objects of anxiety was a beast. This noisy animal 'was' the father, who made so much noise in the adjoining bedroom. Gerald wanted to go in there to 'castrate, kill and blind the father', fearing he would be treated in the same way by the animal. Some of his passing gestures were seen in analysis to represent attempts to fight off the attacking beast.

2 *The evidence that very young children develop a precocious and pronounced*

super-ego (1927a). This position contrasts with that of Anna Freud, who held that the super-ego was weak in children, since they are subject to the influence of their parents. She also argued that the super-ego developed only after the dissolution of the Oedipus complex. Klein observed that play clearly revealed very primitive phantasies. For the child, the analysis lessened the super-ego and reduced the feelings of persecution and guilt. Rita assumed the role of a cruel, punitive mother towards a child, represented by a doll or by Melanie Klein herself. She was the victim of fears and guilt feelings and felt the need to be punished (Klein 1926b). Further analysis of little girls (1928) also showed that the principal source of anxiety linked to femininity was the fear of the mother's retaliation against the girl's body in response to imagined attacks on and despoiling of the mother's. Klein also noted that these anxieties were mixed with feelings of guilt and depression. She stressed that the tendency towards reparation was an essential characteristic of mental life (1927b, 1934). She observed in Trude (3 years and 3 months old) the oral-sadistic and sado-urethral root of aggressive impulses. She compared the analysis of a paranoid girl, Erna, with that of other less afflicted children and adults, which led her to hypothesize that anxieties of a psychotic nature belong to the normal development of children (Klein 1926b, 1929).

3 *The formation of split figures, one persecutory and the other idealized*, also with regard to the analyst.

4 *The antedating of the Oedipus complex* (1928, 1945).

5 *The early development of transference in children* and the need to interpret it immediately. For example, when Rita enters the room she is quiet and anxious and asks Klein if she can go out into the garden. Klein follows her, but immediately interprets the negative transference. The girl comes back into the room relieved.

It was the observation of children in the analytic relationship that led Klein to postulate the existence of *internal objects*. She noted that there was no correlation between the often destructive images of the mother, as they appeared in play, and the behaviour of the mother in reality. These images emerge from within the child, and the parental imago, that is, the relationship with the internal phantasy figure, is transferred onto the analyst. On this point Segal (1979) comments that just as Freud's study of adult neurosis led him to discover the child in the adult, so Klein's study of children revealed the infant in the child.

Klein observed violent defence mechanisms, active before repression. The child carries out violent expulsions and projections to free himself from internal persecutors and from his own sadism. The principal anxieties afflicting children are fears of persecution, linked to the mother's body and the father's penis, and the defence systems are varied, including splitting, idealization, and phantasies of restitution and reparation.

Child neurosis was considered a defence against underlying psychotic anxieties. Thus for Rita, or for Erna, obsessive rituals served to placate complex anxieties of a psychotic nature. Segal (1979) points out that in her observation of children Klein noted that object relations, both with real objects and especially with objects of phantasy, were operative as far back as observation is possible, and that the primitive part-object relations played a leading role in the structuring of internal objects, the super-ego and the phantasy life of the child.

Klein also stressed that the child's unconscious phantasy is precocious and omnipresent and has an influence on his every perception and relationship. This attention to the unconscious phantasy led to changes in the concept of symbolism (1926a, 1930). Thus symbolic meaning underlies not only play but all the child's activities, such as reading, writing and performance at school.

The analysis of psychotics began with the case of Dick (Klein 1930) and the reflections on symbolism which followed. Klein observed that since the child desires to destroy the organs (penis, vagina, breast) which stand for objects, he imagines the objects as threatening. This anxiety contributes to making him equate these organs with other things, which in turn become new sources of anxiety. In this way the child is forced to establish new equations, thus laying the foundations for his interest in new objects and creating the conditions for the development of symbolism (Klein 1930). (It was Dick's terrible anxiety about the fantasized attacks on his mother that caused him to lose all interest in his mother's body and in anything that symbolized it.)

The most primitive phantasies are not verbal in nature. Initially they are related to the body, then they are visual, and finally they can be expressed in words. Sometimes verbalized phantasies may reveal those of an earlier developmental stage. Isaacs (1948), for example, reports the case of a girl who, at 20 months, was terrorized by one of her mother's shoes that had a broken sole. Fifteen months later she asked about the shoe, adding: 'It was going to eat me.'

The libidinal phantasy of a good, nourishing breast is reinforced by positive experiences, while negative experiences reinforce the child's phantasies of bad objects. Phantasies can also ignore reality, and the suckling baby afflicted by persecutory anxieties may reject the breast his mother offers him, as has been observed in babies suffering from eating difficulties. This conception of unconscious phantasy is connected to the idea that, at birth, there is an ego capable of establishing rudimentary object relations which uses primitive psychic mechanisms such as projection, introjection and splitting (Segal 1979).

Observation and interpretation

The child, then, creates distance by means of personification. He represents and governs phantasies which would otherwise be intolerable, masters anxieties and anticipates projects, gives meaning to and organizes his own internal world, metabolizes and orders the stimuli which reach him from the external (and internal) world, and learns to control phantasies and impulses.

All this can be observed and can become the object of study and reflection. This has been shown in large part thanks to the method of infant and child observation proposed by Bick (1964) and developed by Harris (1987), Meltzer and the British school,[4] among others.

I find it rather limiting, however, that there has been a prevalence of studies on the relationship between infant and mother, whereas less attention has been directed to all the other situations in the child's life and the no less important relationships both inside and outside the family.

Moreover, I feel that insufficient study has been devoted to the interference which the presence of the observer, however neutral he may be, causes in the field which he himself helps to create. Indeed, if we hold that there is an interplay of projective identifications, there can be no neutral presence, no presence that does not have multiple effects on the field. Advances are made in the study of the child in the family context when, in observing the infant, adequate account is taken of the group function and of the observer's influence on the structuring of the relationships in the family. Bick was aware of this (Magagna 1987), but she did not revise the concept of neutrality with sufficient theoretical elaboration (Vallino Macciò *et al.* 1990). Furthermore, the extension of the observation of children to other contexts with appropriate settings and modalities (hospitals, kindergartens, nursery schools, daycare centres, etc.) entails assessing, from a psychoanalytic point of view, the entire range of situations which the child may experience, as well as other relationships he has outside the family.

In any case, everything that is observed becomes the property of the observer and the object of study for the group that works on the observations, though it cannot be communicated to the parents because of the specific situation. The parents may receive indirect benefit, however, through the way in which the observer presents himself and participates.

What makes it possible and legitimate for the observer to 'interpret' or rather to propose a meaning for play, is the establishment of a *setting* and a *contract* (albeit with the parents). Only this act creates a shared therapeutic relationship. This complicates matters considerably, because from this point on we are no longer dealing with a child playing *a game* (except as an abstract defence mechanism) but rather 'play' acquires full membership in the field. As the interchange of projective identifications creates an emotional fabric common to the couple, the child will use play to begin to narrate from his point of view what is going on in the emotional field. Initially this vertex will be as yet unknown to us. We will have to reach it in order to 'be in unison' with the patient (Bion), to search together and find another vertex that can be shared by both members of the pair.

It does not really matter who expresses the phantasies of the couple while playing. Play is none other than a narration, albeit in a special language, of the emotions present in the room, using characters which may or may not be anthropomorphic. Indeed, animals, toy cars and blocks can all at different times function as 'characters in the session'. What the child continually describes to us is how he experiences our emotional presence, our oral communications, and how we contribute to determining the emotions.

Of course – and I never tire of stressing this – *this is a listening vertex which must oscillate together with the others*: i.e. that which regards play as an expression of phantasies of the internal world and that which sees play as reflecting external and historical facts.

The vertex that is relevant to us, however, focuses attention particularly on the functioning of the couple. This is because the child's mental phenomena enter the field, in part through the projective identifications in the analyst's mind. Like the analyst, the child will react, accepting or rejecting them, and thus contribute to the constitution of the specific and unrepeatable history of that particular couple. In this sense, as we have already mentioned, there is a continuous oscillation between the transferences (understood as repetition and as outward projection of the phantasies of the internal world) and the relationship (understood as the new 'couple-specific' situation). This oscillation is produced by the encounter of the two minds and gives birth to a unique, new story capable of reorganizing the old ones, which are saturated and waiting to be thought about (Bezoari and Ferro 1991b).

It should be underlined that this oscillation is never-ending, and in this oscillation the transference is no less important than the paranoid-schizoid position in its oscillation with the depressive position (PS$\longleftrightarrow$D). It is precisely the paranoid-schizoid position and the transference that constitute the source that feeds any creative process, provided there is re-elaboration in the relationship and in the depressive position. In play, too, the characters of the session should be regarded as 'functional aggregates', before their meaning (symbolic, relational, functional) can become explicit. In other words, they emerge from the daydream that the patient continually puts forward as alpha function is stimulated by the encounter of the two minds and by the reciprocal anxieties and defences.

The notion of the functional aggregate allows us to suspend judgement on whether what is proposed belongs to this or that member of the couple and permits us to 'play' with the characters and consider them nodes which facilitate the growth of narrations. Ultimately, it makes no sense to decode symbols or 'true' meanings which are often intolerable for the other member. Our aim should be to increase the capacity for thought and the expansion of the mind (Tagliacozzo 1982).

Of course, the characters of a game can be viewed from other vertices, as representatives of the external world (the father or mother, a brother or sister). This vantage point focuses greater attention on the conflicts, emotions, thoughts and affects which involve 'those' real characters, which is what is generally considered in structural models. At the same time the characters in a game reflect the inhabitants of the internal world, the internal whole objects or part-objects, and the unconscious phantasies which enter the scene as externalizations of these internal realms. Here we have a Kleinian point of view.

In the model which I consider unsaturated and relational, a vertex which oscillates with the others, the characters of the session, as they appear in play, represent the affective holograms of the couple. They speak above all about the mental functioning of a particular couple, at a particular moment, about the communication or lack of it which is taking place, and about what can gradually be thought about and elucidated.

Play and the analytic relationship

Play, then, can be regarded as the way in which the child continually signals from his vertex what is happening in the field, what defences are being activated and when dysfunctions and breakdowns in communication occur. This vantage point allows us to use these signals to get through to the patient.

This is not very different from how we think about a dream, even an adult's dream. Play is simply a dream which is unfolding before our very eyes and continually changing according to where we are situated and how we intervene, or how we do not intervene. From a field perspective, regardless of the stance we adopt, we always enter the field and modify or rather structure it.

I have always found it a useful exercise to ask myself how a child's play could be converted into an adult's dream, or how the dream of an adult might be translated into the language of a child at play. Take for example a child who runs around the consulting room, strikes the keys of a typewriter and complains that it does not work. 'It's electric, and it's not plugged in', answers the therapist. Here the child is signalling that he is not receiving adequate responses, that touching the 'keys' has no effect and that the 'keys' do not activate reverie. There is a tense, electric situation which induces the therapist to 'pull out the plug' so that he is unable to give even those mechanical responses which would normally be sufficient to satisfy the 'electric' child.

The child wants to communicate and he sends out a signal that a response is not forthcoming. There is an electric tension of underlying emotions, and a defence mechanism is activated. Pulling out the plug which reflects the therapist's defence in the field may, from the child's intrapsychic point of view, be an inducement for him to do the same, to become absent, not to respond to the electric emotions he is faced with.

An adult's dream might correspond almost image for image to such a game. For example: 'I went to the office, sat down at the typewriter and struck the keys, but nothing happened . . . a thunder storm had blown the fuses, etc.'

A child continually reveals the mental functioning of the couple. An example taken from the analysis of Carlo illustrates this point. Whenever Carlo feels that the therapist's mind is withdrawing and becoming unavailable, that it no longer receives his projective identifications because it can no longer tolerate the pain linked with the extremely primitive anxieties the analyst must face, he picks up a block, goes to the wall and starts hammering on it. Then he glues the block to the wall, signalling that the therapist's mind, to which he adheres, has become impervious. He starts to play again only when the therapist, with Carlo's help, manages to establish contact with her own unavailability. In this way it is not only Carlo but the couple which oscillates between moments of two-dimensional functioning with adhesive identifications and moments in which the relationship becomes three-dimensional and the projective identifications can function once again (Bick 1968; Gaburri and Ferro, 1988).

When a child begins to play, for example, 'Davide takes the animals out of the box, the tiger attacks the lion and the dog defends the lion', we have two options. One is that of grasping the relational meaning, in terms of emotions and feelings, and proposing it to the child. In this case we observe that we are immediately faced with anger and aggression but we also point out that the person being attacked needs to be protected. We can ask ourselves what has happened – why there is so much anger, but also concern. In this way we render the feelings evoked increasingly explicit in the transference. But there is another more complex approach, especially with children who work fast. In this case we leave the child's 'denominations' as they are, participate in the game and offer interpretations on the basis of the characters proposed by the child. In this way we build up a story together, turning our minds into the stage on which the story will be enacted, though we must never lose touch with the relational meaning of what is happening. Here, then, we comment on *the tiger's* anger and on *the dog's* concern for and friendship with *the lion*. We allow the story to develop without decoding excessively, which would merely risk obstructing the unfolding of meaning.

Let me give another example. If a child switches an electric heater on or off, we do not necessarily have to interpret this gesture. We can try to understand the function of regulating the heat that the child feels he requires, and we can strive to interpret the need for this 'heat' in order to clarify the game for him. But if we stopped here, we would simply be avoiding the problem. The child must for once be granted the ($\male$ $\female$) *realization* of that need he felt by making available to him the therapist's own capacity to regulate the distance and to provide him with more heat. This can be achieved by lowering defences and offering the child the warm, sharing mind he needs in such a way that the interpretations do not appear to be a defence against emotional experiences and so that the child is able to realize fully that intimate, passionate, emotional meeting which is, as Bion says, the analytic encounter.

An adult might say: 'I was driving the car . . . There was a young woman with me who shared the expenses. There was a man who never shared expenses and always kept his distance. Once, when he was asked about his lack of concern for a friend who was in trouble, he said that his grandfather had lived to be a hundred years old because he always minded his own business.' This could be a formulation in adult language of what the child is doing while playing. That is to say, it would be a description of our defences, of our lack of participation or our withdrawal, our defending ourselves from a more exposed and dangerous contact (which shortens life!). We would have to 'work' this description in the countertransference. It would certainly be of no use to interpret the patient's fear, since this would merely expose the wound rather than heal it. We would then have to find the capacity to establish contact and reduce distance, fully aware that we cannot know, in terms of the field, to what extent the distance we had created was our defence and to what extent it derived from something that was activated inside us because we assumed the patient's projective identifications, transmitting 'distance and non-involvement'. However, it is only by accepting the defences of the field as our own that we can transform them.

When we are dealing with play (and I am still speaking about play in the session, as otherwise we would not have the right to 'interpret' a child's play), if we seek to construct a shared story, we must maintain contact with different levels of interpretation, many of which will remain silent in our mind. One of these is historical. This is the reformulation of a past experience, or a current experience in the external world, which strives through play to be rendered less frightening, more manageable and, finally, metabolized. Another level is the one I would call intrapsychic. Here play shows us which phantasies the child is involved in at a given moment, for example, which internal mother he is dealing with. This level is *transferential*, that is, the child uses his projections to make a sort of film of his present affective story and uses us as a blank screen.

There is still another level which I consider the most important and particularly worthy of our attention (indeed the others may be taken for granted). This is the *unsaturated relational level*. Here play truly becomes 'our shared story'. We are continually taken to task for what we are, how we interact, how we defend ourselves or participate. Here we have the possibility of adopting a vertex which allows us to consider play as a narration of what the child feels is happening in the couple. The difficulty is to accept that this account speaks about 'us' and not about the child's repetitions or projections. I would now like to present some clinical illustrations of these different models of listening.

The need for narration: Marta's tree

What was said about 'weak' interpretations and the construction of a story shared with the patient, as opposed to the unambiguous extraction of meanings, is also applicable to play. This is shown by Marta's drawing (Figure 3.1). Marta is an 11-year-old girl whose analysis had come to an impasse, in the face of strong, unambiguous interpretations which made her dream about not being received following her 'own *intervento*'. Here she was referring to a surgical operation ['intervento'] she was due to undergo, but at the same time communicating the fear that her oral communication ['intervento'] was being dissected rather than received in all its textual richness. The analysis began to bloom again, like the tree on the right in the drawing, when I managed to give up searching for strong, unambiguous meanings.

Play, beta-elements and the formation of the container

Let us recall for a moment the example of Renato's little bison (Chapter 2) in order to point out which characteristics differentiate the Kleinian model from that inspired by Bion, as Lussana shows (1991). Lussana stresses the unsaturated construction of the Bionian approach as opposed to the saturated interpretation proposed by Klein and points out the importance Bion assigns to 'gathering, containing and digesting emotional experience . . . rather than raising unconscious phantasies to consciousness'. This issue has also been addressed by Speziale Bagliacca (1991) (Vallino Macciò 1992) who emphasizes the need for oscillation between the activities of containment and interpretation.

Mental space: a problem concerning the transference of the relationship?

The diagnostic observation of Andrea, a 6-year-old boy, taught me a lot. I learned how important it is for a child to have someone next to him with

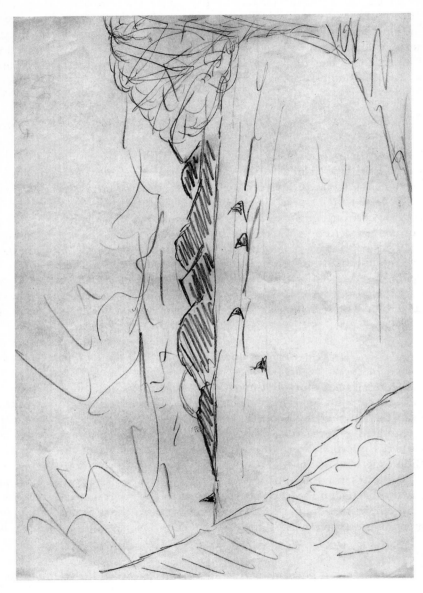

Figure 3.1

available mental space. It is not necessary to understand him, but the analyst should have the availability that allows the child to feel that whoever is with him has a mind, a capacity to receive him, to think and to delay.

For the sake of brevity, I will present only a few flashes from the sessions with Andrea. The mother tells me that Andrea cannot stand carrying any weight, not only in a figurative sense, but even literally. Let's say a coat or any other object; he immediately gives it to his mother. The mother, for her part, has no one with whom to share her own burden: 'My husband is very reserved and doesn't want to hear about problems', she says. Consequently, she has to search for unreflected, acted out solutions in order to unload her weight anxiety. So when Andrea starts elementary school and tells her that the teacher is too demanding and that he has no friends among his classmates, the mother immediately suggests that he change schools. Andrea breaks out in tears. He had no intention of changing schools. How could she say such a thing? 'I had found a solution for him', is her observation. This mother cannot think, she cannot wait; unable to take problems upon herself she tries to solve them immediately.

Let's look at a few extracts from the observation of Andrea and see how illuminating it is, even though it is shorn of the connections and bridges of the original context.

Andrea speaks about his mother who is in the waiting room. He says that she will feel as though she were suffocating because there are no *windows*. Later he says that he will come back, if I put in a window.

Andrea builds a house with wooden blocks. A hippopotamus attacks the house and manages to make a crack in it. But he is angry and disappointed, because the house is full of bricks. 'There's no space . . . this is a trick', he says and destroys the house.

He begins a drawing depicting a boy who has found refuge inside a grotto with a tiny entrance hole. He makes it even smaller so that grown-ups cannot come in. There is an opening through which his mother, who has 'an arm in place of her head', searches for him but of course with no success.

During the observation Andrea says: 'Who knows whether I fell on the floor, when I was born and came out of Mummy's belly?'

'If a 6-year-old got into Mummy's belly, she would explode. If I had to get into Mummy's belly, I would have to cut myself up into pieces to make myself small enough. How would I become big again? I'd have to sew myself back together.'

The game continues: 'There's a boy in a boat and he has to sell everything there is in the boat.' (He takes apart all the pieces inside the boat he has built with blocks.) 'In exchange for these things, which he gives up, they give him a cow, a big male cow, a little boy cow.'

It seems to me that Andrea gives a good explanation of the lack of eyes that look, understand, provide light and illuminate meaning: the 'windows' he talks about. He describes his mother's mind as 'full up'. It is impossible to enter, and even if you enter there is no space, because it is full of bricks (the hippopotamus, angry Andrea and the house). Then there is the drawing (Figure 3.2) in which the mother has no 'head' or mind, but rather an arm, a muscle with no internal space, a mother who does not think. Andrea's drama is that he must break himself up in pieces in the hope that some piece might find a place inside his mother ('I wouldn't fit whole, Mum would explode'). He must mutilate himself, give up parts of himself, which are then sold off, split, in order to obtain a family (the cow, the big male cow, the little boy cow). The fundamental question Andrea might ask is this: 'When I was born, was there someone there, was there a mind to receive me, to think about me, to give meaning to all the nonsense that surrounded me?'

If priority is given to the relationship rather than to the transference, further levels of meaning open up which can be more easily shared: Andrea's fear stemming from the awareness that he is being 'observed', while awaiting an answer; the fact that this waiting, this examination, makes him feel as if he were waiting, suffocated; and the idea that he will return if I become available to give him mental space and therapy (windows).

There is a fear, which increases as Andrea waits for my judgement, that I might reject him, that I might not be available. (In fact, I was asking myself whether I had room for him in my group of patients.) When my interpretations focus on internal objects rather than on the real problem of whether I have room for him, Andrea seeks refuge in the tiny opening, in my meagre availability at the outset, in which I awkwardly search for him without devoting sufficient thought to what our problem in the field is, since I am caught up in the task of assessing 'his' problem.

Then there is the question: 'And now that I'm here, he'll drop me. There won't be any follow-up to our meeting.' And there is the fear that for me, for my availability, he is too big, too great a burden, so that he almost 'has to' dose himself out in small pieces in order to be taken in. And he seems prepared to do anything, to give up anything, just to be accepted into analysis.

The first level of interpretation is more neutral and we are less involved. At the second level, on the other hand, we speak as much about ourselves, about our emotional availability, as about the patient, and this is far more difficult to accept.

Relationship or field: Claudia

I see Claudia, a 10-year-old girl, after an interview with the parents. They tell me that their daughter is quite backward at school and that she has already

Figure 3.2

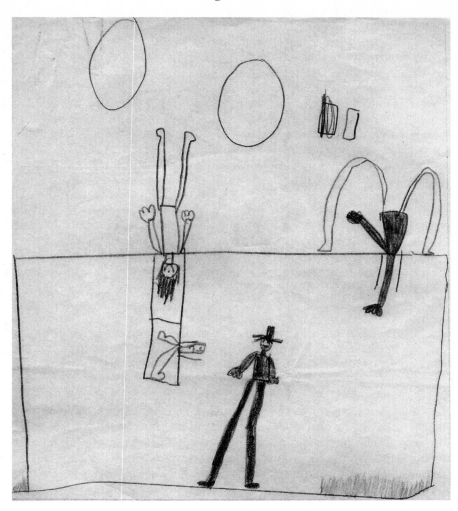

been diagnosed as having a serious mental handicap. Her difficulties with arithmetic seem to be insurmountable, because she cannot understand quantities. She is a twin and for a long time she was kept in an incubator. They show me one of Claudia's drawings. There are two little flowers, drawn in a very childish manner, with much of the stem in common. I think about the problem of quantities: one or two?

Claudia comes to the consulting rooms with her mother, who remains in the waiting room. She suddenly goes to the playroom. There are some things

71

on the table; she looks at me without any expression on her face. I try to alleviate what I suppose might be her anxiety, her fear. But I can't wait to see if she will do something, and what she will do. I can't wait and try to understand, so I ask her if she would like to do a drawing. She makes some totally incomprehensible scribbles. She doesn't speak to me but goes on drawing in the same way for the whole hour.

I haven't understood anything. I'm tempted to conclude that Claudia is severely handicapped. That way, even before being looked into, the problem would be solved for everyone. But I realize that I'm not thinking, that I too have been filled with a great, incomprehensible feeling of urgency, including the urgency to communicate all this to the parents. I realize that I might try to connect my state of mind with Claudia's. I tell myself that I must learn to wait, to be able to observe Claudia again without preconceptions, without feeling the need to give answers. I must try to watch Claudia with the eyes of someone who knows nothing about her, and see if I can give meaning to what she produces, while keeping in mind what I felt after our first meeting: the feeling of not having understood, not having thought, haste.

We come to the second meeting. I have tried to shelve what I know about Claudia and prepare myself for a meeting with a girl I have never met. Claudia arrives with her mother, who asks if she can come back after the hour is over. Claudia goes into the playroom. She is alarmed, frightened. I ask her if she is afraid to be alone with me. She smiles faintly and heads towards the table. Then she sits down. I manage to wait. She picks up the wooden blocks and builds something she says is 'a bridge'. Then she builds another thing: 'it's a house'. And something else: 'a house with a fence round it'.

I say that the bridge makes me think of a wish to get in touch with me, and the house with the fence suggests that maybe she feels like a prisoner in the room. She confirms and does her first drawing, saying it's an abstract picture. I suggest that there seems to be a girl there who is then rubbed out. She seems to be interested and, hurriedly again, makes the second drawing, which she says depicts 'some rectangles with something around them'. Immediately afterwards, the third picture: initially it looks like a house; then she puts something like bars in the windows. Then she quickly scribbles all over the drawing until it is unintelligible.

I suggest that we look at the drawings. I say that the third one seems to be a house with bars: a prison. And perhaps there is an angry girl who wants to erase everything. Claudia goes back to the blocks and makes 'a house with a tree'. (I think she feels I am close to her.) Immediately afterwards she constructs something like an empty cube with some smaller cubes in it. I say that maybe it's a 'mother with some children inside' and that perhaps she is feeling understood. She says that this is true. Then she stacks some other blocks. I say that reminds me of the second drawing, of people who want to be together, next to each other. She seems to confirm this.

She picks up the crayons (and once again I am unable to wait, to tolerate uncertainty, to give Claudia time), and I ask her if she wants to draw. Frantically she begins to draw the fourth picture; it is structureless, incomprehensible. But at this point I think I have understood. I say that maybe she has always felt that others have pressured her, that they have always made her do things in a hurry, as if they never had enough patience. They always ask too much of her and she feels as though she were being chased. That is why she does meaningless things, like the fourth drawing, because she hasn't been given time to think.

Claudia is convinced and relieved. She begins to speak and tells me that that's exactly how she feels, at home and at school. And that's how she felt with me a moment ago. She begins the fifth drawing, this time structured, with two human figures side by side. She tells me about her life at home, and later she tells me that she wants to come back to see me.

I was quite surprised in the course of this session by the variety of possible meanings that could be formulated, by the intense expression of feelings. I was witnessing Claudia's rich internal world unfolding, and this became possible when I showed her that I was able to wait and that I was open to whatever might happen in our relationship here and now. It was precisely at the moment when I realized that I had been unable to wait, the crucial moment of the session, that I understood what was happening to the girl: Claudia picks up the crayons – 'Do you want to draw?' – The invitation is felt as a threat/imposition/injunction/persecution. When she felt persecuted, Claudia could not think, so she did the fourth drawing, 'meaningless, or like a turtle withdrawing into its shell'. When I understood this and made it clear, Claudia responded with a fifth, structured drawing, in which she was once again able to think and symbolize. She felt that someone understood this dramatic experience of internal persecution/enforced haste/a request so pressing that she was unable to think. All this corresponds in part to the hyper-stimulations by which she felt bombarded and to the demands of her parents: the haste, the inability to think and to understand, which I had adopted as my own after our first meeting.

The description I have given of how that first meeting went with Claudia offers matter for reflection. First of all, we should note how the patient's problem has to become the problem of the couple. This occurs when my lack of restraint signals my successful adoption of the fact that Claudia's emotional states are uncontainable. The problem must then be worked through by the analyst before it can be expressed in words, or 'realized' (Bion), as a new kind of relationship with the child. The child, in turn, can then adopt the new way of relating that she has been shown, and experience it directly.

Second, nowadays I am less prone to render meanings explicit (note Claudia's observation: 'abstract drawing'). I would try to stick closer to a text that could be shared with Claudia, striving not so much to extract meanings as to construct a story together with her. It was I, after all, who 'barred' communication and contributed to rubbing out the girl with my hurry to provide an answer. Even then, however, using a different model, more relational than field oriented, I could still grasp Claudia's problem.

The ant's feelers and the urologist's needle: working through and transformation

At the beginning of a session Francesco, who has been in analysis for several years, tells me that he tried to shove the door open several times with his shoulder. Then he tells me about an origami figure of an ant on which he has not yet put the feelers, because he is not sure whether, according to 'the revised rules of origami, in addition to the classic folding and the new licence to cut, we are also allowed to use glue'. Then he talks to me about farm chickens going towards the food and wild chickens running away from it.

Shielded from the wealth of emotional content in Francesco's communication (his fear of my being unavailable, his ambivalence towards the analysis, the transformations underway inside him, his new capacity for separation and his potential regarding the link and reparation, etc.), I pick up a drawing from a previous session in which each of three neighbours is represented with separate paths to their houses, so that each can avoid meeting the others. In this way I take him back to something he was striving to overcome, this side of the Oedipus conflict. Cocooned from Francesco's search for the new, I explain what kind of communication is implied in pushing with shoulders, the ant's feelers, and the non-communicative isolation of neighbours. In my cocoon, instead of sharing with him the impact of his growing, I talk to him about psychoanalysis.

Francesco, in reply, makes an aeroplane and lets it fly, saying that it doesn't take off properly. He tries again and says 'it must be the heavy nose cone weighing it down'. And anyway, the plane looks like 'a plucked bird'. I am not yet ready, however, to grasp the sense of Francesco's words as a comment on my own inadequate interpretation: 'What you're saying just doesn't hold up. There's too much theoretical deadweight in it. It's only a plucked interpretation.' Instead, I head, though cautiously, down the path of possible sexual meanings.

My projective identifications had begun when I used a drawing from a previous session to speak to 'the patient from the day before'. They had evacuated all Francesco's tensions and developments and continued when I denied the meaning of his answer/comment (the plucked bird). And they culminated in the series of questions on sexuality which in reality not only bar the door but also 'discharge anxiety'.

Figure 3.3

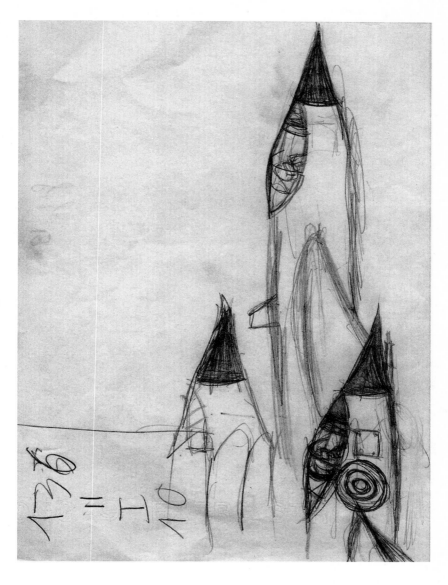

After giving me some evasive responses, Francesco says that he has to go to the urologist for an X-ray, and to do this he has to have a liquid injected into his veins; they are going to use a large syringe with a slender needle. I finally understand that this is how my questions are felt: as injections which serve to have a 'scientific' look inside. In the meantime he has sharpened his pencil and drawn two pointed shapes very close to each other. These become two jets or two guns (Figure 3.3). Finally, once I have grasped that my words are perceived as menacing, they become 'two Italian planes with identifying marks'.

One might think that we were dealing with the most primitive anxiety in the relationship with the breasts, which, once sharpened, rip open, and bombard and drown with milk, rather than feed. But I couldn't help wondering whether this image was taking shape there, at that moment, precisely because shortly before (and during the rest of the session) there was a dysfunction or an inversion of the analytic function: not an analyst receiving and absorbing what is new and changing but someone clogged up who is discharging his own tensions; not an analyst feeding farm hens, but one who is intrusive toward the hen, making it wild. The inversion was directed towards a patient who, rather than feeling improved, felt intruded upon. I believe that the drawing should be seen not so much as connected with the breast but as capable of grasping, in its successive transformations, what was happening then and there between the two minds.

Admittedly, in a field-oriented view, it was necessary for someone to become the vector both of the 'deafness to listening' and of the persecution which activated every attempt to find space inside Francesco to receive the interpretations – Francesco, who was struggling against the doors he found closed to his communications. But allowing the problem to enter the field is the first step towards being able to work with it and towards recognizing that the cycle is the root of every possibility of transformation (Figure 3.4)

Figure 3.4

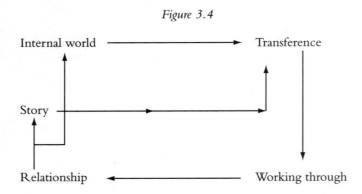

4

Dreams

Dreams are the best proof that mental phenomena in children and adults are essentially identical. In this chapter, therefore, we shall examine the dreams of children, adolescents and adults.

It would be interesting to trace the development of the theory and clinical use of dreams from the beginning of psychoanalysis to the present day. One could begin with Freud's *The Interpretation of Dreams* (1899) and draw examples from the lucid chapter on dreams in Musatti's *Trattato di Psicoanalisi* (1949) in which dreams are 'worked out' according to the principles of Freud. One could then pass on to the Kleinian model to reveal and clarify underlying phantasies. Then there is Rosenfeld (1987), who (explicitly citing Langs) shows how the problems of communication between analyst and patient are often clarified specifically in dreams, and Meltzer, who provides some wonderful illustrations of how the analyst's countertransference and reverie can serve to interpret dreams, as in the fine example of the 'submarine', an extremely clear example presented by Meltzer in *Tentativo di costruire una teoria del sogno che serva per l'uso nella stanza di consultazione* [An attempt to establish a theory of dreams which can be used in the consulting room], a booklet from the Centro Milanese di Psicoanalisi. One would also have to review the latest developments in Meltzer's work (1984) which are the fruit of his contact with Bion's original and revolutionary ideas concerning dream life. For Bion, in fact, dream life is a 'theatre for the generating of meaning', following the assumption that the external world is meaningless until meaning is generated and made usable. As Baruzzi (1989) puts it: 'The analyst weaves the patient's dream material creatively; he does not interpret, but helps the patient, in the highly emotional experience of working with dreams, to complete a transformation from one symbolic form to another.'

Some views on dreams

Theories and models of dreams are like the rungs of a continually extending ladder. Each rung is added to a previous one, and each affords different, but equally valid, vertices and views.

Dreams are able to gather together and make visible moods and emotions which cannot yet be thought about. This operation may be performed in various ways and with different measures of success. Dreams can express a genuine poetry of the mind (Sharpe 1937), or a religion of the mind (Mancia 1987), or they can constitute a forest inhabited by phantasy in its enigmatic state (Resnik 1982).

Of course, it is impossible to lay down all the possible rules for the interpretation of dreams. The classic mechanisms (displacement/condensation/symbol formation/censorship), though revolutionary discoveries at the time, are only some of the possible 'figures of speech' that can be used to create 'the poetry of the mind'; to these Sharpe adds metaphor, alliteration, onomatopoeia, etc. It may be a useful exercise to identify them, but this would be like carrying out the structural analysis of a text.

Several considerations must be kept in mind when 'reading' a dream. It has to be completed by the interpreter's dreaming about it (Meltzer 1984). He must come into close contact with the dream, redreaming and reorganizing it in his own way. His role in the process may be more modest than that of the original dreamer, but it is no less significant.

At an initial level we might say that the patient is the 'director' who films a mass of emotional situations, and the analyst is the 'film editor' who gives order and meaning to these scenes. This is true only in part, of course, because the analyst does not limit himself to editing but also introduces images that have been activated in his reverie. These images draw their inspiration from the communication of the dream, as the receptive, resonant analyst listens 'without memory or desire'. Phantasies, memories, and especially images are set in motion inside him. All this must be organized, communicated to the patient, and reorganized until it becomes a shared story.

Once a relationship comes into existence, one vertex available to us is that which assumes that a dream cannot be regarded merely as the dream of *one mind about itself*, since the projective identifications of the couple structure the common pool of emotions and, I would add, moods. This is the pool from which the dream draws, and to this common matrix it must be returned.

It is useful to interpret dreams in terms of codes. (What was alive yesterday but is no longer today becomes a code, just as what is alive today will be a code tomorrow.)

A structural model of interpretation will account for what have become classic rules and furnish a map of primal phantasies which can then be

78

described to the patient. One drawback of this approach, however, is that the interpretation will inevitably have the flavour of an essay on the patient. A Kleinian model, on the other hand, will help reveal unconscious bodily phantasies, part-objects, and so on.

Such approaches permit the patient to learn more about himself, but as they are based on the idea that therapy serves to render conscious what is unconscious or to bring together split parts, etc., they do not focus on the capacity to transform and think about what previously had no place to be thought about. In other words, they concentrate on *the contents of the mind rather than on the mind itself.* They do not account for the need to transform and expand the mind (a process which presupposes the capacity to think and transform), and on occasion even to construct it. A useful indicator of the fertility of an analytic couple is, I believe, the extent to which the patient's images can be transformed on the basis of the interaction with the analyst: the more different images are created and changed, the more capable the couple is of mobility and creativity.

Seen in these terms, a dream that in some sense draws on the *mental lives of both members of the couple* (and we recall the 'scandal' that Rosenfeld created when he asserted that the patient had the capacity to dream the split-off parts of the analyst) requires a troubadour to compose a song about it and to help weave a story, which can be thought about and narrated, from the syncretic thread of the images of the dream.

We are accustomed to regarding dreams as products of the night's sleep of which they are the guardians, as the working-through of the 'day residues', or as the revelation that the internal world is full of unconscious phantasies.

Bion proposes a radical change in thinking. For him the dream is a bridge between dream thoughts and the capacity to think (Bezoari and Ferro 1998). Bion (1962) also describes the *'dream thought in waking life'*, of which clinical evidence is detailed below (dream flashes in waking life), an expression of the work which the alpha function performs as it continuously transforms beta-elements. These elements arrive from all the accessible and traversable sensorial and emotional channels, in relationship with our bodies, with what we have not thought about, in relationship with others and with the world. The dream thought in waking life is like the Krebs cycle (a sequence of metabolic reactions in the living organism in which chemical substances are transformed into energy for storage in phosphate bonds). Its continuous activity permits the metabolization of ketone bodies (beta-elements). Contact with this dream-like thought is the basis for *reverie*, for deep phantasies of a sensorial, visual or auditory nature, in all the various creative manifestations. This becomes evident when dream images escape from the mental container and appear as flashes in waking life, situated midway between dream and hallucination. Like dreams, these flashes manifest worked through dream thought, but in contrast they lie outside the mind and are visible in the external world. Like hallucinations they lie 'outside' mental space, but are distinct from them because the contents of hallucinations appear like evacuations of beta-elements, bizarre objects, 'nonthought', and are of no use in the construction of meanings. The dream and its communication always represent an important moment. They constitute an invitation to enter a more intimate area of the relationship and to render it explicit. It is like receiving an invitation to peep into even the most secret drawers. I point this out in order to stress the discretion that must be exercised compared with other types of communication. In other words, dreams cannot be read with an 'interpretive picklock', as this would be an improper invasion of private space. There is no question that what our eye allows us to see *beyond the text* is of considerable value to us, but we must respect intimacy and defences. What is lost in terms of reduced communication and shared knowledge about something is abundantly compensated for by the affect of the patient, who feels respected and not intruded upon, and by the progressive introjection of a non-intrusive relationship mode.

Dreams can be considered along a temporal axis, with the aim of grasping certain important structural transformations (for example, dreams which restate the terms of a problem in progressively modified form). They can also be viewed along an axis which reflects the *development* of work (and not the documentation of work completed) in its main function of communicating – in the hope that the interlocutor will pick up on what is happening in the encounter between the two mental lives, between the internal groups, the defences and the reciprocal identifications. Dreams constitute, moreover, a sort of map of how all these things went in the last encounter (especially in the case of a dream communicated at the beginning of a session) or how they are going at the moment at which the dream is communicated.

Bion (1987) says that he would resort to a theory only if he felt tired, and if he felt he had not understood anything of what the patient was telling him. If this maxim is valid for everything the patient says, it is especially true for the report of dreams, that is, when the patient opens herself up completely to communicate with us. Indeed it would be truly disrespectful to approach her while hiding in the protective cage of our theories. Such cages, especially as regards dreams, are plentiful. The greatest risks derive from unilateral, symbolic interpretations, in which the patient's (presumed) symbols are decoded without sharing in the process of symbolization. The patient, in fact, has no 'symbol' to be interpreted. Rather, the process of symbolization arises from the encounter between patient and analyst, as the creation of a new meaning (Meltzer 1981a, 1984; Ferro *et al.* 1986a, b).

For example, Carla, a 12-year-old girl, relates a dream at the beginning of a session in which she was in a house supported on two pillars. From the house she could see two white mountains. As she looked at the mountains she watched a landslide, first with enthusiasm, then with terror. A little puppy she was holding risked being suffocated. Of course, one is tempted not to think about the dream, not to work it over, but to decode it on the basis of an already extant system of symbols. In this way, however, we would deny the girl the specific encounter of two minds: of those two minds, at that particular moment (Leonardi 1987). One might say, in an interpretation that considered only the patient and her internal world, that there is a girl held in the house-arms of her mother with long pillar-legs, who looks with admiration and then with terror at the two mountain-breasts which fill her with milk, and that she feels suffocated when her admiration turns into anger and envy. All this, I believe, would merely serve to make the patient feel alone, and perhaps desperate and guilty, while relieving us of our responsibility: 'I'm not involved with what is happening to you.'

The patient would benefit more from an analyst who thought, one who, let's say, regarded the dream as a precious indication of what the girl experienced in the last session or at the moment immediately preceding the account of the dream, as if she were saying: 'You are flooding me with what you're saying. You risk suffocating my newborn thoughts (the puppy). Slow down.'

This point of view will raise questions in the countertransference as well. There will be doubts about how the interpretations are being regulated with the patient. The analyst will recognize his own lack of interpretive restraint and will wonder whether this was caused by his taking on the projective identifications of the girl's incontinent functioning. But in this way the dream is not viewed as the destination of a situation which requires decoding but simply as the point of departure for further thoughts, some of which may be shared with the patient. These thoughts will then, in turn, activate other thoughts in the couple, making it possible to construct a story together, even a story which results in a capacity to contain, though this may not necessarily have to be made explicit.

There is no truth about the patient to be discovered, but rather truth concerning the functioning of the two minds in the session which must be constructed. Just as in Conrad's *The Secret Sharer*, as Gaburri (1987) reminds us, the patient will be the one to allow us to keep track of what is going on, with his 'toss of the hat'. In our case, the hat that the patient tosses in our direction is his communication, in whatever way it is expressed. In any event it reaches us. If we listen to his continuous narration of where we are and where the couple is going, the patient will help us avoid running aground on the rocks of non-communication. We depend on the patient, our coxswain, and must put absolute trust in his signals, and he depends on us, not merely because we have the nautical maps but also because we are constantly charting our course as we proceed with him.

81

Moreover, I do not believe that the patient should be continually prodded with requests for associations as this is the legacy of a model which holds that the dream already has a meaning to discover. I would suggest that the patient might make associations occasionally, and I would consider as 'associations' everything he said before, everything he says afterwards and whatever comes into our minds, as well as the emotional atmosphere at that moment (Vallino Macciò 1990). This way I have a living, authentic text, which is not considered a text to interpret but a narration to develop creatively and jointly.

Seen from this angle, the dream is a narrative and relational truth about the couple, or better about the mental functioning of the couple. Borrowing from Bion, we could say that it becomes a private myth of the couple.

As Meltzer (1984) points out, not all dreams are equally successful. But the success of a dream does not depend only on the dreamer. The dreamer may, to a greater or lesser extent, construct a poetic vision of what is happening at the depths of the mind, or better, of the relationship. The question is how much poetry (that is, reverie) and how much dreamed material the other mind, i.e. the analyst's, is able to contribute.

Ultimately, the patient's dream constitutes the first stage in the organization of something which has yet to be communicated, and only what comes from the other mind will make the couple's dream complete.

Dream and narration

As I have said, there are many possible vertices in the interpretation of a dream. I would now like to discuss dream as the initial organization of 'moods', of emotions which the couple cannot think about as they have yet to be narrated and shared. 'Characters' are dealt with in some detail in Chapter 5. In dreams, too, we find that the characters can be variously interpreted in terms of their historical reference (historical childhood experiences), their reference to the internal world and its events (unconscious phantasies, relationships with and between internal objects), and their constituting 'affective holograms' of the couple at work (Ferro 1991). These holograms can also be regarded as the syncretic naming of emotions in search of (not necessarily anthropomorphic) characters that will make narrative development possible.

I do not believe that we can speak of the complete interpretation of a dream, but rather of continual rearrangements and meanings which, using the dream as a starting point, can be constructed and shared as an expansion of what is thinkable.

Since there is no truth to discover, except a relational and affective truth, what counts, more than any sort of decoding, is that the analyst be in unison with the patient. He must go and meet him on his own grounds under conditions that the patient can tolerate.

We shall now consider several dreams, not so as to attempt an interpretation, but to suggest possible readings for each, or readings actually proposed in real situations. Of course, the dreams will be presented in terms that will help clarify the vantage point adopted in each case, although in theory one dream would suffice to illustrate all possible vantage points.

The dream and relational vectors of the field: the cheetah and Dingo

I said that a dream can be considered not only as an initial collection of emotions and moods circulating in images, and therefore as the fruit of an initial intrapsychic elaboration of the events of the couple, but also as the draft of a screenplay for which the set design and characters have yet to be developed. But how does this come about?

Gianni, a 13-year-old boy, fills the session with jokes, quips and games, making it difficult to establish any other kind of communication. He is also afraid that his silence, or the things he says, may be communicated to his parents.

One day he shows me some scars he has on his leg and he tells me that he had a dream: 'There was a school . . . a strange animal came out of it . . . a big cheetah . . . the cheetah chased me . . . I ran away . . . the cheetah tried to bite me . . . There were two lions behind bars . . . then the cheetah again . . . I was in the cellar and there was Dingo, my dog, who risked being torn to pieces . . . I tried to wall up the cheetah . . . but then it came to life again . . . and ran after me.'

What can we do with this dream? Of course, at a structural level it is rather clear. It speaks about aggressive, violent parts (the cheetah and the lion) which are feared and split, kept in the cellar, which he tries to brick up, but they come back to life and attack the more affectionate, though wild, parts, perhaps because they have been abandoned (Dingo).

But what is the point of this sort of interpretation? How could it be useful? Perhaps the parts could be distributed in such a way that we accept those which are more persecutory and difficult for us, so as not to let the patient mobilize excessive defences or guilt feelings, and to show how these parts can be recognized and accepted.

It might be sensible, then, and especially acceptable to the patient, to propose this type of reading: Gianni wonders what a strange animal, or strange person, the analyst in front of him is, how much he should fear him, perhaps that he will tell his parents; how dangerous this person is, who can hurt him through the things he says or the way he acts; maybe this is what happens hidden down there in the cellar; upstairs there are jokes and quips which are the bars that keep out the cheetah, a danger he tries to keep under control, but then it comes back to life.

This interpretation allows us to talk about the terrible things that occur in the couple, but in a form that can be received and that does not activate further persecution feelings.

There are elements that suggest other narrations, such as the wounds, or the dingo (the Australian wild dog whose wildness comes from its being abandoned). On this view, the patient's dream is already in the depressive position with respect to the elaboration of anxieties in the paranoid–schizoid position, whereas the dream related by the analyst is in the paranoid–schizoid position awaiting transformation into depressive position; it is non-saturated, waiting to be worked on, transformed, narrated.

But perhaps we can go further and ask whether the dream does not provide material for the working-through. Can the 'cheetah' be worked through and transformed inside the analyst's mind? And isn't it true that the dreamed of cheetah reflects an analyst with teeth and claws, if observed from a vertex and with a sensitivity hidden from us? And isn't the way to achieve unison with the patient to go to the place where 'cheetahs' materialize?

If we consider dreams from this point of view, our task is not that of *taking on a part*, but rather that of recognizing what we are really like when seen from a vantage point unknown to us, until we are finally able to share it.

The field, then, encompasses many possible relational vectors which await possible narration (live, violent feelings; aggressiveness and defences; violent projective identifications and tendencies towards lethargy; the container unsuited to holding excessively intense feelings; an interpretive activity which scratches, etc.). These range from considering the patient's point of view as a projection, to regarding the dream as a description of what is going on between the two minds at a particular moment, thus leaving the characters 'cheetah' and 'Dingo' non-saturated, 'bricking them up' until they become part of a microstory in the here and now. What counts in these narrations is showing the patient the quality, use and elaboration of the material produced in the dream. This makes available a model of functioning which can be introjected (since only in this way can we offer the possibility of introjecting and fortifying the alpha function), where the vector will be chosen according to the story that awaits narration.

The absent character: Carla's lice

Carla is a young adolescent. At the conclusion of a rather uneventful session she expresses a desire for something that might remove the anxiety that troubles her. Then at the following session she relates this dream: she discovers that she has lice and has to shampoo her hair frequently to get rid of them. Carla has a phobia about dirt and always cleans away whatever crowds her mentally. She spontaneously associates the dream with the fact that she often cleans her dog of parasites.

The first interpretation I propose is routine. While she is under the impression that everything is clean and orderly, the dream reminds her that there are anxieties she would like to free herself of, to wash away. It is as if they were stuck to her head, without being expressed and formulated in words. Her desire is simply to free herself of them. My words achieve no effect, or rather the effect is persecutory: 'I feel scolded because I don't talk enough, because I'm not doing the best I can.'

Making use of these words, and of my own sense of dissatisfaction, I present the dream in these terms (thinking also of the 'lacklustre' preceding session): in the last session I was not able to clean away her anxieties, so she was left with the burdensome task of cleaning herself. This has a totally different effect and activates further communications on the part of the patient.

But there is another level: we can consider the dream as an accurate expression of what the patient felt was happening. In the previous session I had actually not been able to metabolize and transform her anxieties, thus leaving her the chore of worrying about the parasites by herself.

The key character lay outside the dream, and though all the facts were there, as in Poe's hidden letter, I was the one who had to find it.

The dream that probes beyond the symptom: Luigi's cleaning alcohol

Eleven-year-old Luigi shows serious signs of anorexia and a phobia about dirt that compels him to go through extensive cleaning rituals involving his body and especially his bedroom. The cleaning rituals occupy a considerable amount of his time: diluted alcohol and detergents are used to scrub the bathtub, the tabletop, the wardrobe, etc., to get rid of every last 'spot of grease'. Every morning before going to school even the insides of his shoes are sprayed with alcohol.

In the analysis he has considerable difficulty coming into contact with the 'root' of all this. If on occasion we manage to find a trace of the emotion that 'dirties' Luigi's spotlessness (Luigi is always the first in the class), it is immediately cleaned up. In the session he plays very little and talks very little about what happens at school, and we do not get far with a direct interpretation of this method of keeping me away from any possible emotional and relational contact. All this continues at length until a dream opens up a different world. Luigi has the dream shortly before leaving on a school trip. (He tells me, with complete indifference, that the trip will cause us to miss a week of work just before the Easter break.) There was a classmate at school who was hitting him on the head with a bludgeon, so Luigi grabbed him, spun him round and made him hit his head repeatedly on the ground . . . His sister had an accident, and some of her vital organs were taken out, although it seemed that she would survive . . . then her house was taken away from her.

The dream allows us to see how disturbing even this reduced interpretive activity was for Luigi (the blows on the head), the rage that was kindled inside him, his revenge (and I now understood the reason for the times when I suddenly lowered my level of attention, and even dozed off for a moment), and the pain caused by missing sessions and the analysis.

The dream opened up the path to the 'unbelievable world', which was continually and carefully cleaned up, the world Luigi called 'the unbelievable world of the other points of view'.

This reading of the dream also made it possible to consider Luigi's symptom in relative and relational terms. I understood that what was for me a minimal activity of interpretation from Luigi's point of view was too intense, violent and dangerous, to the point where he felt he had to disarm me. This understanding allowed me to gauge my interpretive activity better and to avoid leaving him alone with his symptoms. I could now link these symptoms to something, to myself and to the disturbance which I caused him, as with the alcohol in the shoes, which could now be thought of as a way of cleansing all those feelings which the separation activated.

The dream as a narrative, relational truth of the mental functioning of the couple: Emanuele and 'the inseparables'

Emanuele, who had begun analysis at the age of 11, after six years relates a dream in which he went to have a chat with the owner of the local tobacco shop. He adds that he *really did this*, and that it was just a way of allowing another boy to steal the sunflowers, so they could use the seeds to feed two parrots, called 'the inseparables', that he kept in a cage at home.

Rather than thinking of a subtext to reveal, we may consider this a simple description, obtained with manifest content (Torras de Bea and Rallo Romero 1986), of what was *actually* happening in the consulting room in the course of this long, slow march, which in this period had practically come to a halt. There seems to be a session and a chat with the tobacconist; in reality the aim was to procure food, illegally, for the boy's plan to continue the analysis for ever (the two permanently caged parrots that protect each other from conflict and loss, in a twin relationship).

But Emanuele has another dream. A young woman had sexual problems with her husband. Someone, when asked for advice, suggested that she put on more erotic underwear, but the husband was entirely indifferent to the problem. He was only interested in the woman's bottom, a perfect cushion to sit on. He remembers that he had had a sexual relationship with the woman, at her request. But he was young. He gave her his penis, but only in exchange for her bottom. Then he tells about having listened to a splendid duet from Mozart's *Don Giovanni*, and in particular 'In Italy six hundred and forty . . . in Germany two hundred and thirty-one . . . but in Spain already one thousand and three.'

Once again there is no need here for an 'interpreter', but rather for someone who can gather the fruit of the patient's labour. He is not interested in a good relationship, a fertile relationship that produces affects. Our relationship is not like that of the two parrots in the cage, but like an idealized, wonderful duet from *Don Giovanni*. Emanuele is interested in the 'bottom', the 'cushion', the conquest and the relaxation of another session, and yet another, without anything happening. And like Don Giovanni he counts the sessions that take place on X street, on Y street (the various addresses of my consulting room as they change over the years).

Emanuele is interested in looking backwards, to the past, to his childhood. Don Giovanni has only a penis. He is only a boy who is afraid of losing his mother, a boy who day after day renews his denial of time, death and separation. The only thing that lifts him up is sterile conquest, which must remain 'sterile' in order to mark time. In other words, he must continually deceive both the analyst and himself, purchasing smoke from the tobacconist he lives with. The elaboration of these dreams, and of the underlying impasse (Maldonado 1984, 1987), makes it possible for us to resume our progress.

The dream and interpretive modulation: the flock and the donkey

One problem we have to deal with is that of providing the nutrition that the mind needs for its development, following the indications given by the patient. Here we might recall the gastronomic metaphor used by Bion (1987) to describe the activity of the mind; nutritional factors should be supplied in careful, patient doses.

In one session with Carlo, I had been very cautious about decoding meanings, as I was afraid that a strong, unequivocal explication might obstruct the formation of other meanings. In one dream there was a sparrow, and Carlo's fear of finding something warm next to him, the fear of the heat of animals. Then there were memories, which had never been communicated, of positive experiences with various animals. (Up to that point Carlo had been phobic about contact with any sort of animal and, clearly, about his and my animal parts.) At the end of the hour he tells me that an important role in the *flock* is played by the donkey. The donkey follows the flock, and as the little lambs are born they are put into its saddlebags. That way the flock doesn't have to stop, time and time again, so it covers more ground more quickly. I feel satisfied at the end of the session. Then I begin to wonder whether I left Carlo's narrative *too non-saturated*.

At the next session Carlo tells me that he was disappointed because his mother didn't give him a present. Then he tells me that his mother has a heart problem, a first degree atrioventricular block. Nothing to worry about, but she had to have an echography. Then he relates the following dreams: a man in a pastry shop, contrary to his expectations, gave him only tiny slices of cake. Then he took a trip on a flying carpet which, to tell the truth, wasn't Persian or even particularly sturdy. It was just a mat, not very big, but solid in the front. Actually it was a bit flimsy, and he was afraid he might fall into a sea where there were 'crags'.

This time I can pick up on the fear that I may have supplied inadequate answers to his long, detailed oral communication, and that I intentionally passed over certain 'craggy' issues, like those concerning his emerging sexuality, which are also an expression of a fuller and more passionate emotional involvement in his relationships, including his relationship with me.

I do not believe that there is such a thing as a right interpretation. We embark on a long journey, marked by continual adjustments of bearings, by trial and error. It is the procedure that charts the course of a continuously oscillating voyage.

The patient's dream activated by the mental functioning of the analyst: loss of sanctity

A young patient, Marcella, signals to me that my mental presence has diminished. She does this by means of a dream in which a friend she is studying with unexpectedly goes on holiday, leaving her with a heavy workload. The situation becomes intense when she gets violently angry with her mother because she doesn't help her with her homework. Since the patient is in an advanced stage of analysis, I decide to communicate to her that there actually was a temporary decline in my 'mental presence', which she had perceived and signalled by means of her dream.

She is relieved and, once she feels that I am far more present, though still distracted on occasion, she relates a dream in which a strong, robust bare-chested man had lost his halo. A rubber band was pulling one of his nipples so much that he was pulled away. In her dream, she hoped that everything would soon return to its place and that the rubber band would dissolve.

It seems to me that Marcella is communicating that the idealization of the analyst has been undermined (the loss of the halo which had been attributed to me for a long time) and that my mind is once again almost entirely present. At the same time, however, she points out that my attention is occasionally distracted by something which calls it away, but then it returns. Leaving aside other possible meanings, the dream appears to provide a snapshot of the relationship as it is at the moment, also highlighting my own emotional movements. Later we will find that other dreams indicate that our functioning has become good and normal once again.

In looking at the situation in this way, it is not my intention to show that the analyst is guilty, or to discover the *primum movens*. In other words, I would avoid deciding whether the patient's excessive projective identifications caused the analyst to disappear, or whether it was the analyst who had an emotional block. The point is that the model of the field allows us to focus on a problem which the couple is having at a particular moment and to search for a solution in the relational here and now.

The polysemy of dreams: before Jean Valjean

As already stated, every interpretation of a dream is possible. I would agree with Umberto Eco (1990) that the limit of interpretation lies in its economy and especially, I would add, in the patient's right to hear what is most useful to him.

Mario, to whom we will return in the context of hallucinations, is now able to dream. He has a dream in which he goes to see a girl 'not because she has trousers and T-shirts for sale, but for the girl herself. He kisses her breasts, but they're small. Then he goes for her bottom and tries to stick it into her, but he can't get it in. So he steals the money from the cash drawer and runs away.'

He adds spontaneously that 'Pinuccia, a girl he likes a lot, is a bit available, but not too much so. The presence of Pinuccia's boyfriend makes it difficult to get to her, and he feels the angry desire to "ram it up the boyfriend's arse" and steal Pinuccia from him.'

This dream leads inevitably to several considerations: the obvious Oedipal level, the Oedipal aspect of the relationship with me, and the level of part-objects and part-functions. But in addition to these aspects it is even more important for the couple to consider the functions and functioning of the minds in the session, which receive pictorial expression through the characters. It is as though Mario were saying that he comes to the session not expecting to receive clothed interpretations (trousers and T-shirt), but rather those loaded with expectations about the specificity of the encounter (Leonardi 1987). He feels that I am available, but not as much as he would like. So he has to force the resisting container (not sufficiently ♀, but ♂ with ♂) until he creates a situation which is unreceptive to the urgency of his projective identifications. This is what brings him to hate my insufficiently receptive functioning.

What is obtained by forcing a container which is not adequately available can be compared to 'theft', that is, the unlawful removal of something which is considered not to be one's own by right, even if it is merely attention or availability. This is quite different from what happens to Jean Valjean, for whom it is the 'gift' of something unexpected and not his by right which makes it possible to find a remedy for the pain of transformation. And it is of Jean Valjean that Mario is to give me a moving account later when he is met by a mind which is fully receptive.

The dream and the fragility of the container: when a CD is not enough

Mario, now in an advanced stage in the analysis, has a dream in which he was calmly going to a prostitute who lived on the top floor, when suddenly he met a violent man who started to chase after him and managed to find him wherever he tried to hide. Since the dream came after a session in which I had applied some interpretive pressure, I suggest what seems to me to be the most obvious reading: Mario felt assaulted and threatened by my insistent manner. The patient says 'no', and adds that he makes all the schoolmates that bother him (i.e. my interpretations) go away.

Then he tells me that his mother gave him a record yesterday. But she really did it for herself, not for him, just to show how well she could pick out a record. When she asked him if he liked it, he said 'no'. Then he talks about the pop singer, Ornella Vanoni, and how she puts on airs, she's stuck up, never satisfied, she has a house that doesn't have any 'doors'. He goes on to talk about an innocent little girl who *died from suffocation*.

The interpretations that the patient perceives as narcissistic/Ornella Vanoni/without doors *kill innocent girls* (♀) that is, containers which are still fragile, still in the process of being formed. These fragile people cannot come into contact with prostitutes (routine interpretive activity/ the record) or with violent individuals (the analyst who cannot tolerate the pain of containing and of working through but comes out with persecutory interpretations). But this is also Mario's problem, since previously he evacuated in hallucinations what his thought could not tolerate.

The communication as a 'dream' of two minds in the here and now

Luciano, a boy with a severe disorder, begins the session by telling me about his weekend. After a short while I feel totally jammed up inside and have difficulty following him. (I am sufficiently present to realize that he is filling me up with the anxieties that he has accumulated over the weekend.) I feel that I'm not going to be able to keep up with the urgency of his increasingly rapid speech.

At this point he changes direction, sliding over to a branch of the main account, and says that he met a boy who was trying to hitchhike. Someone picked him up, but after a short distance they tip him out of the car and beat him up. (I realize that the part of his projective identifications which has not been received has boomeranged and turned into not only repudiation but even violence.)

I talk to him about his expectations for our meeting, the disappointment, and the pain at seeing me blocked and no longer able to follow him. He listens and then picks up saying that he saw a pretty girl at the discotheque (pretty, I tell myself, just like my interpretation seemed to him). But there were some boys with her, and he didn't know whether he could trust them or not. (So the interpretation was pretty, but dangerous too. He is thinking, 'What will I say next?')

This clinical fragment illustrates how the continuous 'dream thought in waking life' allows the minds to use the various characters that enter the field to tell each other about the changes in their deepest and most unconscious emotional flow.

The dream and the poor mental functioning of the analyst: Rina's scale

Clearly, it is difficult to present 'pure' situations in the session, that is, situations in which there is no intermixture of dialogue, dreams, drawings and play. In line with the plan of showing how dreams can indicate that the analyst is functioning poorly in the session, I would like to present the case of Rina, a young girl who alternated drawings and dreams to signal when a situation was becoming difficult.

The oscillations of the analyst's mind during the session can create a problem (Ferro 1985d) to which I will return. For the moment let us consider the patient's capacity to make us aware of such problems, which can occasionally even go as far as the poor mental functioning of the analyst (Ferro 1987a, b).

This poor functioning is immediately registered, signalled, and sometimes remedied by patients, within their limits of toleration. If, however, the analyst does not become aware of the problem and take control, it enters the field with increasing violence, to the point where it is likely to interrupt communication and provoke negative therapeutic reactions (Barale and Ferro 1992).

Before this occurs, the work of analysis is interrupted, and this 'microclimate of the session' becomes a problem of the analysis. Only when the 'wound' is healed can progress resume.

Some patients stop dreaming, as if they had closed the watertight bulkheads of their ships; others use their dreams as flags to signal what is happening. Each reacts on the basis of his emotional sensitivity, which is often directly proportionate to his pathology. At the beginning of the analysis patients are particularly worried if they have not yet positively experienced the proper mental functioning of the analyst. This is also the case of patients who in their 'histories' have had early experiences with parents whose anxieties and mental lives they have had to bear. All of these patients pass through their current situations as a re-enactment of the frustrating experiences of their past (Miller 1979).

Whenever I have undergone a period of suffering and emotional blockage, due to an overload of unexpectedly sad experiences in real life whose emotional weight was too much for me to metabolize at that moment, all my patients have responded in different ways. From among the many responses I have chosen to cite Rina's.

Rina is in her first year of analysis. She is perhaps the first in the group of patients to notice that something is not right. She seems to become aware of this in terms of the quantity of anxiety which she felt was absorbed and metabolized before, while later she no longer found the same reception. The situation becomes increasingly intense; so much so that there is a serious risk of breaking off.

She signals this in a series of drawings. One of these (Figure 4.1) is entitled 'The weight of the analyst'. There is a scale and two people with ropes tied around their necks. The situation is one of 'almost no way out'. *If the analyst weighs more than she does with his own anxieties* she will be left suffocating, hanged, and she will not have the air she needs. But the opposite does not seem plausible, i.e. the fear that if she weighs down the analyst with her own anxieties, he will be the one to die. The situation seems to have no way out. It is cleared up when, through a dream in which a wall appears between the analyst and the patient, it becomes possible to say that it is the fulcrum of the scale (the wall in the dream) that separates the members of the couple and impedes communication. The wall is formed by the analyst's lack of availability; he is blocked up and cannot receive the patient's projective identifications in his flooded mind. So, contrary to expectations, he offers her merely interpretations/translations/decipherings which really form a defence against the expansion of the mind and a veritable 'wall' for the patient. We find this idea in Rosenfeld (1987) when he speaks of the need for a correct 'opening up' of the mind before any interpretation is possible.

The 'trick' that Rina uses to ease the situation is to reduce her own for a few sessions by narrating a whole series of superficial events. She communicates this by another drawing (Figure 4.2) in which the message is explicitly written out: 'Back soon'. She indicates the importance of this choice in another drawing (Figure 4.3), entitled 'Skipping analysis'.

Figure 4.1

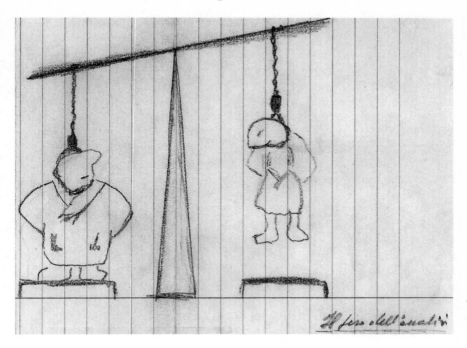

The analyst's underlying mental situation is described in one of Rina's dreams: a man was rushing to dab the wounds of a girl, and perhaps heal them, but he could only use a quarter of the gauze because the other three quarters were already soaked in his own blood.

As the analyst's mental situation gradually improves, Rina dreams about a lift with a broken motor and water flooding into it, but she also dreams of the workmen who are fixing it. Subsequent dreams indicate that the crisis has been overcome.

During this period it was characteristic for Rina to be afraid that she would have to bear the weight of my psychic life (I was her father in the dreams), or, at any rate, she was afraid of being a burden.

My proper functioning resumed when I was able to propose effective interpretations once again, although Rina indicated that she still had some difficulty playing well with Marcella, her best friend, since she seemed to her a bit less inventive than usual. What was missing was the purifying and transforming function of the reverie before each interpretation. 'Narrations' often present the most sophisticated way of expressing this, e.g. the 'fabulous' mother another young patient speaks about, alluding to the mother's ability to tell fables.

Figure 4.2

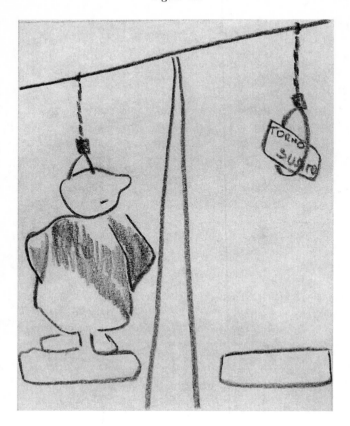

The dream and the vertex of utility: Carmine Manzo

Let us reflect for a moment on the fact that some interpretations of dreams are more useful for resuming proper functioning and activating transformations than others which might be equally 'correct' but could risk worsening the situation of the field. Those which work better seem to involve a transformation inside the analyst's mind, rather than an elucidation or interpretation presented to the patient.

Mario had analysis as a boy. At the time he used to have hallucinations, which were then transformed into dream-like flashes in waking life and finally into dreams. He has come back for some analysis because of deep, unmetabolized mourning at the sudden death of his 27-year-old sister, to whom he was very close.

Figure 4.3

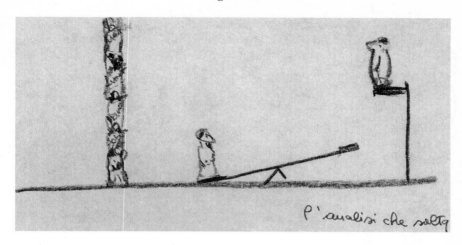

His alpha function must not be overloaded, as it has already been put to a difficult test, and he needs full respect for his narrative text. One day he frightens me when he says that he had the impression that he had 'seen' a thug in his room, a certain Carmine Manzo, Mafia boss and drug pusher. Then he relates two dreams. In one there is a competent mechanic who is fixing his car; in the other, some 'Mongoloid puppets and crooked things'.

My immediate impression is that Mario is experiencing powerful splitting again and that Carmine Manzo is a split-off part of Mario. I had worked on the integration of this splitting for years. But going back to work in the same way will worsen the situation, unless I can tell him that he considers me as a good mechanic when I respect much of what he tells me. If, on the other hand, I say things which I have not thought out enough, if I impulsively say 'crooked things', I end up by 'consolidating' Carmine Manzo, becoming myself the representation in solid form of the stupid bully who can certainly be of no help to him.

Of course, Carmine Manzo also has something to do with Mario, but it is more useful to ask what it is in the analyst's functioning in the consulting room that gives birth to 'Carmine Manzo', rather than to the good mechanic. Only in this way can we bring about transformations in 'Carmine Manzo' and, consequently, in the relationship with the patient.

The dream as feedback: the emperor at the stake

Valentina has been in analysis for three years. After a session in which I come too close to a narcissistic pattern which had been relatively neutralized by then, she dreams about an emperor who was being burned at the stake. At a certain point, however, the emperor got up and walked away, though he was all black from the burns. What was serious, though, was that there was also a little boy there, whom she could see clearly, and he showed no signs of life. His head seemed as if it were underwater. Then she talks about a colleague of her father's, Doctor 'Tarantula', and then of the proverb 'gutta cavat lapidem' [a drop of water wears away stone], and of a snowslide, and about how the snow is not really dangerous, because it makes the field fertile, if it melts drop by drop.

Valentina was providing me with indications about how persecutory, dangerous, and ultimately useless the operation had been in which her narcissistic fabric had been called too deeply into question. The result was, in fact, that new projects, which had yet to be developed, were shaken as well. She was communicating that she had a sensation of risk and suffocation, and that the only way for the narcissistic texture to 'melt' painlessly enough to be tolerated was 'drop by drop'.

Dreams serve not only as feedback, in the terms proposed by Meltzer of speed, distance and temperature, but also as vehicles for transmitting information about the internal world or about ways of coming into contact with it. Most importantly, dreams introduce names and characters which can enter the microstories of narrations and give 'names' to mental and relational facts. The emperor was to become a key character for us and he participated in many stories, often with open-ended, unpredictable plots.

An interpretation which decodes often runs the risk of becoming a parallel text and may even appear in the eyes of the patient as non-affective. In a ♀/♂ coupling, on the other hand, text and story are created together and each member shares almost equally in the narrative-affective construction.

The decoding process also creates a greater illusion of neutrality, or even the illusion that the decoder is not entering the patient's material at all. On the contrary, the analyst enters as a cold, hard, even devastating presence, and, ultimately, the technique serves as a defence against involvement and sharing. For a further discussion on this point I refer the reader to Bezoari and Ferro (1989), in which we describe 'clothed' and 'weak' interpretations. These are a way of keeping the door open to meaning, of presenting oneself in a manner which the patient can accept and, given the unsaturated nature of the inter-pretations, of opening up the path to unpredictable narrative developments.

The dream as a check-up on the analyst's mental life and on the functioning of the couple: Fausta and Marisa

I would like to present a few sketches from sequences which help clarify these points. It is Wednesday morning. Before starting work I receive a communication which causes me some pain and which continues to be present in my mind, though in the background, well into the afternoon, when I have the session with Marisa. The session goes well.

The next day Marisa tells me that she has had a tiring day. A teacher had a sharp pain, not like a pulled muscle but an attack of colic. Then she tells me about a worried mother.

Again on Wednesday Fausta says she would like to 'change offices'. She asks me to answer the questions she puts. (Does this mean that, since I am cluttered up inside, I am less able to answer her emotional needs?) My interpretations are correct, she says, but 'intellectual'.

Thursday: Fausta dreamt that she cried all night because I was with another girl. She begged me to pay attention to her . . . she was afraid that the nuns wouldn't accompany her, that they wouldn't give her a room (my lack of receptivity to her projective identifications?) . . . a clogged sink in which the same things were stirred up.

The patient has the capacity to bring the analyst back into contact with his own mental functioning, and only when this functioning is adequate can the progress of the ♀/♂ encounter be resumed. The journey may be interrupted once again, though, by −K, which often crops up precisely because of inadequate interpretations.

Fausta again, following a session in which I had 'interpreted' correctly, dreamt about a lift that screeched when it went up. Then she found herself in a beautiful room in the company of a hospitable lady. But no one was looking after a little girl, who was suffering a lot and was together with a girl with a plaster cast on her leg. Then she asks me why I'm wearing a tie, and she appears disappointed because I haven't allowed her to change her timetable and now she can't attend Daddy's* lessons.

At this point I can hardly help wondering in what way my interpretation, although correct, was inadequate. The girl suffers because she was 'not accepted' by the rigid girl (interpretation in a plaster cast and a tie). What is the function beyond the interpretation which I did not 'use'? Perhaps preventing the patient from coming into contact with the 'father' function; something which refers to the intimacy of the relationship. Something becomes clear when Fausta relates a dream in which some bread dough goes into a tube and is cut up into many pieces. These pieces, in turn, become 'rolls', but it is the same dough, it did not undergo any transformation. What is it that changes the nature of dough after it has been cut up? The pieces need an 'oven' so they can be baked and transformed, the proximity of emotional warmth.

Marisa, after a session which I considered satisfactory, with well articulated

---

* Translator's note: 'Papi' is the affectionate Italian word for 'father' but also the name of a professor at Pavia University.)

interpretations, relates the following dream: there was an empty cardboard box; it looked like a full wooden box, but actually it was just useless and in the way. (There is certainly envy here, but how was it activated?) I suggest that if the infallible inspector Rock[1] is there (Rock, exciting!/a diamond), he won't let her thoughts develop. She confirms, saying that in the maternity ward newborn babies are stuffed by leaving full bottles propped up in their mouths. Since they are always hungry they become cyanotic. In intensive care, in contrast, the nurses are very good. They pick the babies up to feed them, and they do simple little things with them. Doctor 'DEARSWEET' is there and he is very gentle with them.

The patient perceives the affective value of approaching 'DEARSWEET', provided we supply the patient with our (theoretical and technical) capacities, or our affective world, our passions and feelings. We must especially have patience, warmth, the capacity to wait, tolerance, narcissistic renunciation, and be able to ask of him the least pain possible to realize the indispensable transformations.

Reveries in the session

The most vivid definition of reverie I have encountered is that given to me by a patient. She knew a girl who, whenever she had a problem, went to talk about it with her father. Her father dreamt about the problem and then used the characters of his own dream to help the girl solve it.

This definition corresponds very well to the key stages of any reverie. One must be emotionally and mentally receptive to the other's communication, including the projective identifications. The alpha function must be activated, as well as dream thoughts in waking life. There must also be a capacity to come into contact with these thoughts at the moment when the received emotional state, now transformed, is given back.

All the work of analysis is based on the analyst's reverie, on his receiving, metabolizing, transforming and rendering thinkable the patient's anxieties and projective identifications. Consequently, there can be no movement in the consulting room which does not involve the analyst's reverie. It is merely an artifice, then, to present illustrations which focus exclusively on reverie.

*Maurizio's fuses**

Maurizio is a very gifted boy who alternates violent emotional explosions with moments in which he seems to break off contact with everything and everyone. Moreover, he has a habit which is quite embarrassing for his parents, given the practical consequences: he has a passion for firecrackers★ and he sets them off in the most unpredictable situations.

From the first sessions it is clear, and this can be communicated, that Maurizio's breaking off contact is a sort of 'circuit breaker' which is activated when he is faced with his explosive feelings, whereas the passion for fireworks is something that allows him to manage, control, and at the same time express this 'explosiveness'. But what allows me to come close to these feelings is the fact that I can speak with him about the various types of firecracker known as 'little kittens', 'big kittens', and 'pirates', and talk about how they are connected with the difficulty of integrating his gentle and affectionate parts (little kittens), his more active and aggressive parts (big kittens), and his predatory and violent parts (the pirates).

The reverie was the moment which made it possible for me to recognize a different vertex from which to narrate what was happening in Maurizio's emotional and relational experience.

The tarantulas, Gregor Samsa and the little chick's heart

Grinberg *et al.* (1975), commenting on Bion, say that a mother with sufficient reverie can intuitively guess the truth about her child's feelings and can return them to him in a form which he can tolerate more easily. But this is also the essence of the process of symbolization, something to do with the movement of emotions and affects, something which involves the analyst's reverie, his receptivity and the patient's feelings, all at the same time.

The interpretation with reverie, that is to say the successful process of symbolization, not only creates new material in the patient but also changes the way in which the patient's mind functions. This is what Rosenfeld (1987) means when he speaks about psychotic patients who, if properly understood, make use of neurotic mechanisms in the session.

But the process of symbolization is continually threatened both by factors which derive from the analyst's internal situation (persecution, $-K$, the paranoid-schizoid$\longleftrightarrow$depressive oscillation) and by what arrives from the patient in terms of primitive mental states. Another factor I would add is the 'refusal' of the analyst's mind to make itself permeable to narratives which are terrifying or evoke excessively painful contacts. In this situation, taking refuge in theories often becomes a successful autistic defence (Alvarez 1985).

I would like to show the capacity for reverie, and with it the possibility of successful symbolization in the session, by drawing on a clinical illustration published in Ferro *et al.* (1986b).

★ Translator's note: 'miccia' = fuse (long or short); 'micetta' = short fuse, fire cracker and kitten; 'micettoni' = bigger bangers/ fire crackers and bigger kittens.

Andrea is in his third year of analysis. He began when he was 7 years old because he had symptoms of anorexia and because of difficulties he had with his classmates. The boy also has serious physical malformations and has undergone plastic surgery on more than one occasion.

Andrea brings some beautiful drawings to the session. In the middle of one there is a big sack made of two sheets of paper glued together on three sides. I ask him what it is. 'Nothing,' he says, 'just a game.'

I am amazed when I realize that the bag is full of hundreds of paper strips with the word 'TARANTULA' written on them in every possible way. I'm speechless. I don't know what to say. But more than one thing comes to mind. Is that how he perceives my words? Or is it anger? An internal world inhabited by spiders? What is the spider a symbol of?

I feel that I am not on the right track. There is something inside me that I can't digest. I have the feeling that I'm blocked up and likely to make myself permeable to something terrible.

We put the bag aside, but even outside the session I find that I am phantasizing about spiders and 'bags full of tarantulas'. 'If Andrea had asked me to put my hand in the bag, and if I had known that there were hundreds of tarantulas in there, I'm sure I would have refused. If, on the other hand, I had not known, I would certainly have pulled my hand out in horror.' The paper tarantulas begin to take shape as *real* tarantulas.

Then I think: 'The difficult thing is for the mind not to withdraw in the face of something horrible (the spiders?). Why would it be strange for the mind to withdraw, if the hand would have withdrawn in horror?' But I can't get any further. More time passes. Then Andrea tells me about some nightmares he had, with spiders, or more specifically 'orpioni',[2] and he explains them to me. He also dreams about caterpillars with wings, 'midway between caterpillars and butterflies' – disgusting animals.

The next session he brings me a paper he wrote in class: a long list of proverbs. He starts reading out the list, and I begin to feel bored. I think: 'That's it. He doesn't want me to speak.' So I distance myself, listening to Andrea's lullaby of proverbs. But many things come to mind, and they begin to find connections (Figure 4.4).

Gregor Samsa comes to mind.[3] I wonder how his mother behaved with Andrea as a little mutilated baby; how receptive she was towards this little spider and those projective identifications which, still under-metabolized, appeared as horrible presences. I wonder how much Andrea has felt that he and his projective identifications have been rejected, even by my mind as it became impervious to the anxieties of transformation, this time in a process moving in the opposite direction from that of Gregor Samsa.

In the meantime Andrea has finished reading his proverbs. Now he tells me about what he studied at school. They did some *tracking* and they studied

Figure 4.4

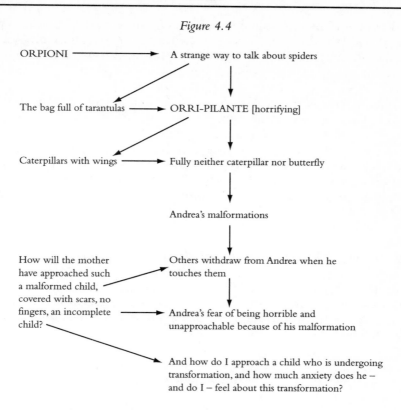

the nutritional value of different foods: carrots, peas, eggs. You need about 2,000 *calories* a day.

He seems to be saying that the heat and intensity of the relationship make it possible to do some 'tracking'. We too are on the track of the anxieties stemming from the changes Andrea is undergoing and which are so frightening for him. At last I can speak to him about the fact that I had taken a long time to understand how frightened he was by the inner changes that were taking place, and how much he sensed my rejection of these anxieties. I often expressed this refusal by seeking refuge in references to the body. His malformations, rather than his fears of emotional change, gradually become active and make him more alive, aware and apparently defenceless. He smiles calmly and says: 'Teacher arrived late at school today.' Then he talks about the cat and the games he plays with it. The cat has grown a lot; it eats everything it is given. It feels lonely when Andrea is away, and now that it understands that it is loved 'he no longer thinks he's of another race: he's beginning to convince himself that he too – the cat, of course – is a person, a human being'.

I do not interpret this communication, as I do not want to expose to too intense a light that something which is taking place to humanize the 'spider' in Gregor Samsa. Here too I am aided by a reverie: I imagine a roll of film which, if exposed to light before fixing, will lose what was being revealed on it.

A few months later, Andrea makes a special REFUSE container with a sheet of paper. In the past, the waste was either left to pollute the toy box or hermetically enclosed in a crunched-up sheet of paper.

There is no longer a closed box with TARANTULAS in it, but rather this open container with no lid (a permeable mind?) which contains refuse, part of which I am asked to dispose of. He tells me he saw a documentary about how chicks are hatched. 'You could see the heart taking shape and begin to beat.'

The pathology of dream function

Let us now examine a variety of phenomena connected with how well the alpha function operates. These range from dream to dream-like flashes in waking life, to transformations in hallucinosis and to true hallucinations (Ferro 1993b).

Hallucinations

Bion (1965, 1967d) regards hallucinations as a mechanism that serves to evacuate anxiety and an excess of unmetabolized emotional stimuli from the mind. It is a mechanism analogous to psychosomatic disturbances and group behaviour 'in basic assumptions'. This evacuation takes place through the sense organs. Their functioning is inverted, as undigested beta–elements are expelled into the external world, along with traces of the ego and super-ego, i.e. fragments of the psyche with which these elements have come into contact, thereby creating bizarre objects. (Imagine a film show being interrupted by a mechanical fault which results in projecting not only bits of the film but also pieces of the crank, lenses and spools of the projector. The viewer has visual experiences which cannot be integrated into the sequence of images he was watching on the screen, and the images become meaningless.)

Of course, hallucinations are always an expression of an extremely serious situation and of the need to evacuate massively in order to avoid even worse situations, such as the confused dream-like situations of the most dramatic psychotic experiences.

Reference to the case of Mario will help distinguish hallucinations from other similar phenomena. Over the years Mario passed through all the stages beginning with the need for massive evacuations and arriving at the full capacity to dream and thus to hold, contain and metabolize in the internal world everything he could not think about before.

Before going into a discussion of the case, I should point out that however we regard hallucination – as the failure of the dream (Bion 1967a), violent destructiveness acted out on thought (Bion 1965, 1967a), defence against annihilation (Aulagnier 1985), lie (Meltzer 1982a, b, c) – it seems to me that it can be brought back to thinkable levels. This requires an intersubjective journey, based not so much on interpretive deciphering as on operations of reverie/transformation. Reverie and transformation must deal not with the content of these hallucinations but with the panic, terror and confusion connected with them.

When Mario comes to analysis, at the age of 11, he is rigid and repressed, and he has a phobia about dirt that forces him to walk with folded arms so as to avoid any possible contact. All this had been desperately and rigidly held in and right at the beginning of the analysis it found somewhere it could be experienced.

At the first session Mario and I were totally unprepared for hallucinations. From the beginning they had no 'name'. They could be described but not named. It took us some time before we could give them a name. It was Mario who said 'allu . . . allu★ . . . alluvioni' ['floods']. In time they became, again in Mario's words, 'the things of the other world'. This occurred when we were already able to manage them better, to avoid being paralysed by them, and we had begun to find a way to use them together. At this point Mario had already become able to distinguish between the hallucination and the external world which we shared. Mario had had to overcome a terrible period in which he was confused about 'what he saw, what was really there and what wasn't' and about 'the problem that certain things were logically not there, and yet they were there'. At the same time I was equally confused because I did not always know how to answer his anxiety-laden questions, which he used to try to orient himself in a universe gone crazy: 'But is that radiator next to me really there or is it a hallucination?'

There was a period of panic and disorientation, in which I believe I took on Mario's panic and disorientation as my own (and I feel that this 'unspoken' part of the relationship is extremely important in Mario's analysis). Then I decided which path to follow: 'Yes, the radiator is really there' (and at the time I was wondering whether this answer was already an acting out!). 'But you are also asking me if it is true that there is someone close to you to help you orientate yourself.'

★ Translator's note: rather than say 'allu . . . cinazione' [hallucination], which is what he really means, he says another word. Compare Chapter 2, p. 37.

I think that then and there both Mario and I appreciated the first part of the interpretation more, as it helped him to distinguish. Today I believe that both of us appreciate the second part just as much, since we then established our permanent working procedure. We have never given it up, even in the most dramatic phases of our long journey together: when Mario 'wasn't asleep, but he wasn't awake', such an anguishing situation that I cannot find words to describe it.

Later the hallucinations became 'the things of the imagination', which could be distinguished from those of reality: 'things that I can see, but that shouldn't be there, things that are out of place'. We learned to treat these things as precious material for us, trying to seize the moment at which they appeared, the sentence that preceded or followed their appearance, the moment of the transference countertransference, and how far they were from the end of the week.

From a field–oriented perspective, hallucination could be considered as that portion of anxiety that needs to be evacuated, as it cannot yet be sufficiently metabolized and transformed by the relationship and by the alpha functions of the two members in the field (Bezoari and Ferro 1990).

Transformations in hallucinosis

Alongside genuine hallucination Bion (1965) describes what he calls 'transformations in hallucinosis'. This phenomenon, like hallucination, is evacuative, but it involves less disintegration of the projected material. Consequently, sensorial elements are expelled but with 'shreds of meaning' attached. The subject, then, perceives around her things which are intrinsically meaningful, without needing, nor being able, to think. In contrast to hallucinations, transformations in hallucinosis entail not the perception of 'objects that do not exist' in external reality, but rather the perception of 'nonexistent relationships' (Meltzer 1986b).

Meltzer (1978) gives a fine illustration of the phenomenon when he describes a child who makes a construction out of Lego blocks and then takes it apart. In the sections that are left intact one can still see meaningful pieces of the project he was working on.

In Mario's analysis this passage was marked by his perception of my feelings and intentions, which were then projected not into the room but directly inside me. There they were perceived with clearly sensorial characteristics, such as the 'terrible rage and fury' directed against him, which he saw in my eyes and which gave him no peace, though he was unable to think about it even for a moment.

We should say at this point that the relationship begins to serve as an adequate container for mental states which are projected and evacuated.

There they find a place where, initially, they can be contained, although they are not yet sufficiently transformable.

Dream-like flashes in waking life

I have already mentioned that dream-like images can be projected outwards, that is, as more elaborated products of the process of the mentalization of experience. This is what Meltzer (1982b) refers to when he describes patients who, as they are speaking, perceive a visual image which commands their attention, without the image bearing the traits of a hallucination. We are dealing with phenomena that lie between the dream and the hallucination, which may be defined as outwardly projected dream-like flashes or images.

The question arises, of course, as to how we can distinguish between hallucinatory phenomena and visual flashes. Meltzer (1982b) states with conviction that if a dream thought with a recognizable meaning can be identified in the image, then we are dealing with a hallucination. He stresses, moreover, that it is not the content of the image which is decisive. What is significant is, on the one hand, the behaviour of the patient, who 'if we are dealing with a dream image, is able to collaborate and give associations, whereas he cannot give associations to a bizarre object'. The other, important distinguishing feature concerns the countertransference of the analyst. In the case of hallucination the analyst is aware that he has lost contact with the patient and with what is happening to him, whereas with the dream-like flash he can develop his own associations and reveries.

Here are a few examples, drawn from the analysis of Mario, of how these 'dream-like flashes in waking life' present themselves. I will begin with a session selected at random from the period I am referring to. It was a phase in which there was good understanding between Mario and me, and there emerged new, at times affectionate, feelings towards me. As I felt authorized by the relaxed atmosphere of the session, I linked up with material he had brought and asked him: 'If Dad wants to now, can he come into the room?' In reply he has a 'vision': 'I see a frog,' he says, staring at a corner of the room.

The same week another patient, who was not psychotic, instead of 'hallucinating' at the idea of something she found disgusting, viz. the idea of having closer contact with me, dreamt about 'a frog in a pool where she had to bathe' and about shuddering at the idea of being touched by it.

I gave Mario an interpretation of what he saw as if it had been a phantasy or a dream: 'You see the frog when I come too close.' He replied that I must tell his Mum and Dad not to come too close to his room.

A few sessions later, when I asked for a fee increase, he saw, in anguish, turds everywhere. I told him that it was 'dirty' for me to ask him for a raise just when he was working so hard to put money together for the holidays; he was afraid that I was insensitive. The vision disappeared before the session was over. The request for a raise made him feel afraid that he could not pay. It represented the analyst's request for additional suffering, which he was not certain he could afford, but he did not feel he had 'the right to eat without paying'.

Still with Mario, before the appearance of genuine dreams, there was a period in which there were frequent dream-like flashes. I recall his 'I see a loaf of bread moving away' at the end of a session, and the return of a dream-like image toward the end of the analysis, when I was 'resisting' this idea – Mario signalled this to me with 'I see a pair of pliers holding me back.'

From the vantage point of field theory, we can say that this phenomenon indicates a full capacity of the minds to metabolize and transform emotions as they are progressively activated, although it is not yet possible to introject a container to 'keep' the dream function in.

I have also come across dream-like flashes in waking life in patients who had not begun with hallucinations. They have always corresponded to the fragility of the container, that is, the incapacity to keep emotions in which are too intense. When I told Carla that the summer holidays were approaching she became frightened and said: 'I see a frog swelling up . . . it's exploding.' Hers was a sort of live coverage of her anxieties of fragmentation. On another occasion she gave visual expression to her disappointment, when an interpretation did not adequately grasp her feelings, by saying: 'I see your chair breaking and falling to the floor.' When she was anxious about the long summer break she saw 'a slithering worm'. This suggested that she felt she would be without legs and flat on the ground during the holidays and that she was not being taken into consideration.

Needless to say, it is essential to distinguish these phenomena from true hallucinations, which reflect a far more serious state not only of containment functions but also of thought itself.

Returning to Mario, dreams began to make their appearance in the analysis after he communicated that the boy who lived downstairs from him had had an operation for hydrocephalus. They stuck a little tube and a little box down his throat to unclog his head. Before, he had been paralysed by all the tension and sometimes he vomited.

Lacking the capacity to dream and an object capable of reverie, the overcrowding of emotions had paralysed him. Now a new situation had been created in which violent sensations and emotions could be channelled into the relationship with me, or contained in dreams, rather than being vomited out in hallucinations. The little box represented, I think, both my mind and the dream, which bore witness to the introjection of a container.

Of course, the raison d'être of dream flashes in waking life can be explained in terms of the concepts introduced by Bion and developed by Meltzer. Meltzer asserts that night dreams, which we may or may not remember when awake, are simply a sample of a continuous process which unfolds both when we are asleep and when we are awake. There is a clear reference here to the alpha function which continually elaborates emotional and sensory experiences, transforming them into elements that can be used in thinking (alpha elements). The dream thoughts about these elements constitute the initial level of aggregation.

Dreaming is a fundamental psychic activity, a veritable matrix of the meaning of each individual's emotional life. From this matrix arise additional forms of more abstract thought and their verbal expressions. This is tantamount to saying that meaning is generated in the psychic dimension of a *theatre of dreams*. There, images and words are integrated into *characters*, and these characters contribute to the creation of narrative *plots* (Bezoari and Ferro 1990).

In concluding this section I would like to recall Bion's (1978, 1980) statement:

> The analysis takes place in the present and can take place only in the present: when people speak about the future, or about what they remember or what they desire, they are speaking about a strong present feeling. We have those desires and those memories in the present, and it is in the present that we live.

It is certainly not a simple matter to embrace this position in its entirety, since we too, like the patient, often need those thermal shields provided by the dislocation in time and space of the events of the session (the story, external reality, recollections, etc.). But the phenomena of hallucinosis, drawings and dreams can help us make Bion's words understandable and part of our experience, since it is easier to consider them immediate expressions of the relationship and the communication. In this sense, dream–like flashes (and their nearest narrative derivatives, which I would call quasi dream–like flashes) bear witness to the entire emotional flow as it develops in the analytic couple. I refer to 'the nearest derivatives of the dream–like flash', because we should not keep different communicative media completely separate. Different ways of communicating must be respected as to their form (anecdotes, dreams, memories, etc.), their levels and splittings, and the patient's capacity to tolerate pain. But the therapist must remain fully aware of how pertinent are the facts of the session and their implications to the relationship. It is this vertex which enables us to trust that psychic facts can change.

A close derivative of the dream in waking life is the visual element, in its central expressions (that is, in the ideal spectrum which ranges from hallucinations $\longleftrightarrow$ transformations in hallucinosis $\longleftrightarrow$ projected dream–like images in waking life $\longleftrightarrow$ dream–like images in mental space $\longleftrightarrow$ visual phantasies). This is why it refers to something more genuine, more meaningful, and thus creates a sort of bridge which can easily be crossed in the relationship with the patient and with ourselves.

These visual elements, which are close to dream thought, facilitate association on the part of the listener. At the same time the 'unplugging' of consciousness allows these flashes to tumble down, as it were, into a sequence (which passes from the visual to the narrative), and it may well be that in this operation lies one of the loci where symbolization can take place.

From this point of view the phenomena of hallucinosis/drawings/dreams represent different moments of transformation processes which are continually taking place.

What are presented here as conclusions, then, could become the point of departure for further reflections concerning the following points:

1   The interpretive activity of the analyst, which occupies a place in a spectrum ranging from *transformations in hallucinosis* (the analyst, suffering from anxieties provoked by the patient's truth and clutching on to his theories, sees relationships which are not there), to *drawings* (partial focalizations of events of the session), to *dreams* about the session (those rare and fortunate occasions when every shred of dream thought finds expression).
2   The metaphorizations of the visual, such as those that appear in the 'visual evocations of the narrative' and in the 'word drawings of the session' – the narrative interpretations.
3   Ways of 'dreaming' about a session, a conversation or a drawing, and then narrating them.
4   The introduction of the concept of the 'functional aggregate' and of features of the character – as defined in Chapter 6 (Bezoari and Ferro 1990; Ferro 1991). These are viewed as holograms of the mental functioning of the couple in the session, that is, as a visual sparked off by the interplay of narrated reciprocal projective identifications.

Countertransference dreams

As Barale and I have argued (Barale and Ferro 1987), countertransference dreams, present in the analysis of both adults and children, are important for various reasons. They certainly make available to waking thought material that would otherwise be difficult to obtain. But even prior to this, it is quite likely that the very fact that they take place constitutes a transformation, reintroducing into the relationship emotional material which has been metabolized, elaborated and enriched.

Reflecting on these dreams may help shed light on two things: first the *internal passage*, that is, the progress which emotions stimulated by the therapeutic encounter go through in the analyst's mind; second, how processes like reception, assimilation, metabolization and the transformation of those emotions are activated in the analyst. Countertransference dreams also reorganize the mental analytic toolbox and the relationships between the internal objects sharing in the dream work. They recreate spaces for reception and symbolization, and restructure the activity of the alpha function (under markedly trying conditions). All these reordering and fine-honing operations do not concern merely the relationship with one particular patient, who may in fact appear in the dream. They often involve groups or clusters of patients or issues, in part raised by patients and in part deriving from the analyst's own mental life. In short, we are dealing with complex muddles which dreams have to untangle.

Countertransference dreams cover the entire range of paranoid–schizoid ←→ depressive position oscillations. They fluctuate in ever-changing ways between functions of reconstruction and enhancement of meanings and functions of evacuation. Most often countertransference dreams occur in circumstances when the analyst is going through a period of suffering or difficulty. Sometimes this is connected to entirely personal affairs, on other occasions to the vicissitudes of the analytic encounter with one or more patients, or to phenomena of projective identifications bombarding the analyst's zones of suffering, or to the very maintenance of the setting.

Countertransference dreams may also be regarded as a sort of analyst's 'safety valve' which serves, under special conditions, to ensure the permeability of the spaces reserved for the capacity to receive and think about the patient's projections. Once again drawing on the paper co-authored by Barale (1987), several functions and categories of countertransference dreams may be distinguished as follows.

The analyst's dreams that shed light on the relationship with the patient

This is the classic use of countertransference dreams, which makes it possible to recover countertransference aspects which are not in contact. A well-known illustration is that given by Winnicott (1949). In the analysis of Mario there was a particularly important dream in which I saw him both as an adult and as a child who was still in need of care. This helped me to get in touch with two different levels of the patient's functioning, neither of which could be excluded in favour of the other.

Dreams that concern the countertransference and the analyst's mental life: untangling and separating

These are dreams which involve not the relationship with a single patient but rather with a group of patients.

Dreams that make it possible to 'restore' the analyst's mind with respect to a group of patients

The analyst's free time (the ten minute break between one patient and another, nights, weekends, holidays) is not as 'free' as it might seem. Dream work bears witness to laborious digestion which, at times, is carried out with a certain amount of suffering. This makes it possible for the analyst to take a difficult but significant step. He can ask himself what these dreams say about his own internal world and which of his own splits they may help him overcome.

At the beginning of the summer holidays I dreamt that my grandmother advised me to scratch a little scab off my nose. Actually, it turned out to be a boil filled with pus. By making a false move, then, one might run the risk of contracting 'cerebral septic venous thrombosis'. But anti-inflammatory or, if necessary, antibiotic drugs allay the danger. One should not underestimate the burden of a year's work. It cannot be scratched away or ignored, as my grandmother suggested, with phrases like 'It's nothing to worry about.' The problem must be recognized and effectively healed, even if it is not serious in itself, but only potentially dangerous. The treatment begins during the holidays, and the anti-inflammatory drugs and the antibiotics may be precisely those dreams which will follow in the summer void; dreams about the more seriously afflicted patients, some evacuative in nature, others more medicinal. It seems that the analytic function never rests. It works to metabolize the depths of the analyst's mind, which finally dreams about 'a disassembled car which he tries to fix as best as he can . . . and he manages to fix it'. At this point, there is no longer need to dream (or to remember dreams), and the vacation begins.

Dreams with greater impact provoked by patients' destructive elements (violent projective identifications from patients activating the analyst's obscure areas)

We are dealing here with dreams which attempt (not always successfully), in emergency situations, to prevent the analyst's mind from 'clogging up'. These are dreams which alleviate mental suffering, by means of the reconstruction of meaning and of symbolic spaces. I dream that I am in Africa and, anticipating that the savages will attack, build some wooden panels to protect me from their arrows. The panels do not seem to be particularly sturdy, though adequate for the purpose. They are tied together but I am afraid they might be too fragile. It occurs to me that they might be more secure if each panel were reinforced with an upright pole.

What is described here is contact with the difficulties at work. There is a protective barrier capable of absorbing. We also have indispensably distanced ourselves from the patient. But there is a need to resort to a paternal function, or to a combined object, which can ensure the analyst remains mentally stable. I believe that the primitives who people these dreams, and their chaotic movements, are connected with the situation that develops when the analyst's mind receives the flow of the patient's projective identifications and accepts the onerous commitment to transform them. But in these circumstances the work which the thought of the dream performs is itself tiring. The analyst's mind is really labouring. The impact with the patient's projective identifications brings into play old scars, blind spots, or even areas which have never been saturated and activated in the internal world of the analyst. This labour consolidates and brings into operation the resistance and quality of the internalized good objects, which are involved in the tiring job of containment, metabolization and transformation (Lussana 1992a). So countertransference dreams have to do with situations of suffering in the analytic relationship (and they create suffering as they unfold), but this suffering may be just a more obvious form of that physiological 'passion' which accompanies the analytic process when genuine transformations take place (Barale and Ferro 1987).

5

The dialogue: characters and narratives

I have postponed discussion of the dialogue to this point because dialogue is constantly present in play, in the relating of dreams, in commenting on drawings and, of course, in verbal interaction. As these modes of expression are tightly interwoven and often overlapping, the description of drawings, dreams, play and dialogues as separate entities is ultimately an artifice to aid clarity of exposition.

On the other hand, just as I find it enlightening to transform a child's communication into adult language and to ask myself how a child might communicate what an adult expresses in words, and vice versa, I feel it is useful to pass from one form of expression to another. In other words, I ask myself how a dialogue might be reformulated as a drawing, how a drawing could be narrated, how a game might appear as a dream or a drawing, and so on. This exercise helps one find more flexible interpretive tools and at the same time confirms the notion of the unity of mental facts. Indeed, it is merely the expressive channels which vary according to the specific needs at any given moment.

Different listening vertices are available when considering the analytic dialogue. It is possible, for example, to focus on the historical, referential level, which provides us with information about a child's external, and affective, reality. What the child tells us, then, allows us to establish contact with his real, external world and with the feelings this world provokes in him.

The child also talks to us about his inner world of phantasy and about the way in which this world enters into relationship with us and with our inner world.

But there is another level that I feel should hold greater interest for us than an interpretive approach focusing on mental structure or on the type of functioning that the child experiences and brings to the surface with us. 'I saw a film where some scientists were slicing up an egg to see what was

112

inside, but that way the chick didn't hatch' is a communication that invites us to think about the obsessive functioning of the child, who, by rationalizing and slicing up the contents, prevents original thoughts and affects from emerging. Considered in the transference it also makes it possible for us, in the child's eyes, to accept responsibility for what happens. In other words, we can suggest an interpretation showing that sometimes we want so much to know and understand that our attempts to clarify his communications and emotional states end up by preventing them from being fully expressed.

There is yet another level, which must be regarded in harmony and in oscillation with the others, which I consider to be the most important specifically for the analytic situation. Here we take the patient's point of view as 'true', a point of view which signals a *functioning of the relational field* in which we are just as involved as he is, and within which the interpretation plays a minor role. Of crucial importance is our capacity to effect a change and a transformation in the way we present ourselves to our patients. This means, returning to the communication mentioned above, that we accept that from the patient's vertex we behave with him (or he with us, it hardly matters!). We are like scientists who actually cut up the communication to show what it is made of, and in this way impede its growth and development. At this point we must change the way we function mentally and interact in the field, so that the field itself can change. The change does not necessarily have to be interpreted. What is important is that our attitude is different from that of 'scientists slicing up an egg'. This becomes possible by going over this 'attitude of scientists' in our working through until it is transformed, let's say, into 'factors that offer food for the growth of chicks'. This is not achieved by means of interpretations, but rather by helping to create the conditions for a new and more fertile mental encounter, by offering a different mind, one that can provide what the chick needs to grow and facilitate an *emotional realization* (♂ ♀) thus far unknown and inaccessible to thought.

Whether and to what extent we are able to carry out this operation is regularly communicated to us by the patient, with the aid of the characters and other communicative means that he (or we) may introduce into the field.

As pointed out in Chapter 1, this approach has much in common with the notion of the field as postulated by the Barangers (1969a, b), by the Barangers with Mom (1983), and by Corrao (1986, 1988). It is especially akin to Bion (1983) when he states that the patient with a serious disorder (I would say the patient's primitive parts) always knows where we are and how we are interacting with him.

From a theoretical standpoint this simply means that there is an alpha function constantly at work, and that dream thoughts in waking life are being continually formed. In particular situations they may escape from the mental container and be projected outwards as dream-like flashes. These are customarily the 'dreamed' response to sense perception stimuli.

Characters, stories and anecdotes belong to this level of communication and constitute a genuine hologram of the deep mental functioning of the couple. This is equivalent to saying, and I never tire of repeating this, that there is a level at which the patient continually dreams and tells stories about us, as we appear to him, from vertices unknown to us. But we must accept this truth, for which we are partly responsible, in order to foster more field transformations. Of course, this level is not exclusive, nor is it one to which we can remain attached. What is important, as Hamon (1972) says, is to ensure that there are many, continually oscillating models.

The emphasis I have laid on 'characters' (which do not necessarily appear in anthropomorphic form in the session) justifies a brief review of how the 'character' is considered in the various narratological models as well as in the different models of the mind. Precisely as it seems to me that a parallel evolution between the two fields of study can be observed.

As to the narratological aspects of the question, we can distinguish between three main groups. In the first I would put all the so-called psychological studies, that is, those that consider the characters in a text as though they were real people with their own depth and individual psychology. So in the text we find events and encounters involving people with their own peculiar characteristics. Characters could be extended on the basis of their individual characteristics. This group includes all idealistic, Romantic, pre-semiotic studies.

The second, very large group emerges with the Russian formalists (Sklovskij 1925; Tomasevskij, 1928; Tynjanon 1965 etc.). These writers overturn the earlier approach, which focused on literary procedures, and in different ways and to varying extents subordinate character to plot. The group includes: Propp (1969, with his interest in the typology of fairy tales); Bremond (1973, who elaborates a code of roles and actions); and the earlier works of Todorov (1965, with his focus on the structure of the tale, how the narrative fits together and how the characters fit into the story). All these writers share an interest in the text itself, which is considered understandable by the objective exploration of a critic standing outside the text.

The third group may be considered those who, though with varying emphases, have stressed the need to take into account the *constant and necessary interrelationship between text and reader*. The principal exponents of this tendency are Eco (1979, 1990), the later works of Todorov (1971, 1975), and Hamon (1972). Hamon sees characters as a construction of the text and as a reconstruction by the reader, and subdivides characters into referential, commutating and anaphoric.

Referential characters are historical, mythological, allegorical or social, and they allude to a complete, fixed meaning. They serve to anchor the narrative, and they ensure 'the effect of reality', as Barthes (1966) puts it. They can be understood in proportion as the 'reader' understands the culture from which they come (e.g. Napoleon, Richelieu, Venus, the knight). Commutating characters signal the presence of the author in the text; they are spokesmen for the author (e.g. the ancient Greek chorus, Doctor Watson beside Sherlock Holmes, any artist character, etc.). Anaphoric characters require a reference to the peculiar system of the work. For the reader, these characters weave into the narrative references and allusions to segments of disjointed utterances. They have an organizing, cohesive function and are the reader's 'mnemotechnic' signs (e.g. confessions, flashbacks, predictions, quotations, etc.). Hamon stresses that each character may belong simultaneously, or alternatively, to more than one of these character types: each unit is functionally multivalent in the context.

Hamon regards the character as a *discontinuous morpheme* and concords with Todorov that the semantic label of the characters is like a construction that is built up piece by piece on the basis of reading time. To varying extents, the character is always a blank space, an 'asemantheme', which cannot be catalogued together with an already given meaning. Only step by step will the reader be able to know the full meaning of a certain name or of a particular character, and the reader himself will contribute to the construction of that meaning.

Semanticization depends on the systematic whole of the story, on the relationship that obtains among all the characters in the story, on the intertextual competence of the reader (Eco 1979), and on the possible worlds that are conjured up in the course of reading (Eco 1989).

In this third group an interesting debate has evolved between supporters of unlimited semiosis and drifting of meaning and those who hold that there is a limit to possible interpretations. These are limited by economy, the nature of the reading process, and the 'rights' of the text (Eco 1990).

We find a similar tripartite evolution in the discussion of characters in psychoanalysis. There is the structural model in its various forms, the Kleinian, and what I would call the 'unsaturated relational model', which I attempt to describe in Chapter 7. (Of course, it is totally artificial to compare such different situations as the analysis of the story and the psychoanalysis. The characteristic of the psychoanalytic situation is that it confronts two living texts which interreact and transform each other.)

In the structural model the characters of a dream, for example, represent a thought or an attitude in a discussion that is taking place in the mind of the patient. The analyst's task is to mediate between the conflicting voices, so that each can be heard. The characters mentioned in the session are those of external reality (referential characters), such as 'the older brother', and are the occasion (or the motive) for expressing conflicts with these figures. They are historical conflicts that can be elaborated and resolved in the transference.

115

The things the patient speaks about, moreover, are not characters in the dialogue but are considered as concrete objects (a watch, for example) around which conflicts erupt and revolve. (In contrast, in the relational model 'gums and teeth' are ways of personifying affects or alluding to emotional phenomena in the consulting room.)

According to the structural model, then, a patient's communication which concerned, say, the non-use of the father's clothes would be regarded as concerning the actual clothing of the actual father and the conflicts with the father which these clothes spark off. They would *not* be thought of as having to do with the way the patient uses or does not use the analyst's words, or with the son function of the field, or with the way of using/not using what comes from the sense-generating (father) function of the field. In other words, they do not refer to the interconnections created by the mental functioning of the couple. That is expressed by means of narrations using (not necessarily anthropomorphic) characters as knots in the net.

In the Kleinian model reference is to the unconscious phantasy underlying the communication, which is confirmed as the real 'hero' in the narratological sense of the main character in terms of emotional weight. In this view the characters of the session are decipherable, not session specific, and correspond to bodily phantasies.

Unconscious phantasies, thus understood, are to be made explicit in the interpretation of the transference. 'Characters' appear in various guises which, once 'decoded', essentially refer to unconscious phantasies. There is no construction of a 'story' but the description and the interpretation of the phantasies 'of the patient'.

The characters of the session, then, may be internal objects of the patient projected onto the analyst, who has little or nothing to do with them, except that he serves as a screen for these projections and acts as decoder/ interpreter, applying a code provided by Kleinian theory.

To illustrate how the model works, and to practise its application on a written text, we might take the beginning of Richard's twenty-sixth session and examine how a character enters the scene and how it is interpreted.

Richard arrives on time for the session. He has two things in his attaché case: a little fleet and some new slippers. This second object in the bag, of which no notice is taken, seems very sweet to me, like a desire for 'home' and a possible substitute for Richard's rubber boots. Certainly, in the pre-ceding session, Klein had interacted with Richard so as to encourage him to open up, as he opens his bag, and to arrange himself both in a position to be able to attack and defend with the fleet, in an attitude of tender familiarity. Then Richard speaks about his mother in bed. (Perhaps he is concerned for Klein, as he shows affectionate apprehension for her: 'It's up to me to do her part.') Referring to the phantasy of flight, he says: 'What a silly idea to run away.' He takes off his boots and lowers his defences.

Klein (who is intent on erecting her ingenious theoretical edifice) seems to be following her own line. She is very active and speaks of three preceding sessions and of sharp pencils. These are all things that were not in the verbal or emotional text of the patient she had in front of her.

Klein insists with active interpretations, and it appears that Richard defends himself by being distracted, listening to the noises in the street. Then he adds that recently, while he was travelling in a bus with his mother, a hostile boy got on and immediately frightened him. It is as if the session could have followed either of two separate paths (or both together), that of the slippers or that of the fleet, but followed only the latter. Indeed attacks are spoken of. But what are we to think of the 'hostile boy'? I believe, as I will explain shortly, that it is an affective hologram of the functioning of the couple and that it belongs neither to one or the other of the pair but rather arises from the encounter. Richard perceived Klein's words as threatening, as issuing from an analyst who was hostile and dressed for battle. In response, hostility towards this attack was activated in him. The fleet has to do with the situation in which one of the two is not willing to listen (not ♀).

Richard is afraid of this climate. The bad boy is the hostility-character-climate function of the couple's interaction/non-interaction. But Klein's interpretation is not 'The bad boys are the words that frightened you' but rather 'You are attacking the unborn children in your mother.' That is to say, Klein interprets the characters of the session as expressions of unconscious phantasies of the patient's inner world. It is as though there were already a text 'inside' the patient waiting to be deciphered. This is partly true, of course. Richard had his past and his phantasies. But when he arrived at the session he was sufficiently unsaturated to permit the construction of different possible stories, depending on how the other interacted.

It is also true that we are dealing with the foundation stones of a model under construction, and it was this model which commanded Klein's attention. She was more didactic in the case of Richard than in the clinical material of, say, *Envy and Gratitude* (1957).

Before continuing I would like to open a brief parenthesis. Why is it that with the Kleinian model we often find so much hostility and persecution in patients? The reason, I believe, is that there had not yet been a reflection, which we owe to Bion, on *where to put the interpretations*. This reflection is necessary if interpretations are not to force, or even break, the mental container in which they are placed. I think that this is one of the most common sources of persecution: the premature forcing of interpretations, which are often correct, into a container which is still inadequate to receive them.

I remember the appreciation a girl expressed for the care with which I made an interpretation adequate and domestic (Richard's slippers). She told me about a trip to China she had taken with her father and about how surprised she was when she saw that, even though China was a world power with weapons and missiles, the shop assistants wrapped packages very carefully, using heavy paper and sturdy string, so they were easy to carry.

Now let us address the unsaturated relational model. In this model the two minds need to tell each other what is happening between them, and especially what is going on at a deep level in the interplay of projective identifications. The characters serve to construct stories, which are developments of the holograms of the couple's functioning. The creation or the presence of characters in the session not only answers deeply felt affective and communicative needs, it is also a function of the defensive structures of the two minds in the session as well as of the possibility of their coupling. Consequently, a story is constructed which is necessary for both minds. It is specific and unrepeatable.

The creative procedure of the analytic dialogue (Nissim Momigliano 1984) is far more complex than that of the narratological relationship between author and reader. The relationships described by Todorov are doubled: author's account/imaginary universe evoked by author/imaginary universe evoked by reader/reader's account. In the dialogue we are faced with two authors who are at the same time readers or, as Nissim Momigliano says, a four-hand sonata in which the (couple's) affective themes are continuously introduced, reintroduced and transformed.

The character takes on particular quality as an affective hologram of one functioning of the couple and is characterized by extreme mobility. The emotions of the couple provide colours and tones, and their words serve to aggregate and organize, so that forms and structures can be derived from them. These affective-narrative figures, which change as the relational structure changes, are the only means the minds have of describing, to themselves and to each other, what is going on between them. The narrations of the couple serve to transform underlying emotions and to make it possible to generate, rather than decode, meaning.

Once again, it is worth recalling that there is no need for the 'character' to assume human or animal form; it can be anything communicated in any way. Doriana, a girl who had been in analysis for some time, responded to an inadequately balanced comment of mine by saying that quite probably she would have to miss a session. A gap had opened up between a tooth and a gum and she would have to undergo a painful operation (missing a session?) in order to bring them back together; otherwise there might be risks (of negative transference, of provoking a negative therapeutic reaction?) (Barale and Ferro 1992). In this case, it is obvious that the tooth and the gum are 'characters' of the session.

Before moving on to illustrations, I would like to mention briefly how the concept of 'functional aggregate' captures this feature of the character as a hologram of the functioning of the couple and give an example of what I mean by 'respecting the textual quality of the patient's communication'.

The textual quality of the interpretation and the narrative transformation of beta-elements

Carla is an adolescent who began analysis because of a narcissistic pathology which was connected with the emergence of anorexia problems. She also had problems of sexual identity. She felt she lacked an internal space and for a long time thought of herself as a boy.

In working with Carla I soon realize that the homosexual friend who appears on the scene signals a male–male [♂ ♂] functioning of our minds in which the projective identifications of one find no space in the other. I am attempting to force interpretations into a container which is not available, since I am unwilling to function in a fully receptive (♀) mode.

For some time I try to adopt a receptive way of listening, remaining close to Carla's text, using the characters that she introduces, and performing a 'weak', unsaturated, measured activity of interpretation.

After years of work (and Carla has by now found a boy with whom her affective and sexual roles are progressively achieving definition), one day she becomes aware of the opening up and the availability of a receptive space inside her. She says that she can no longer tell stories about 'others' in the analysis, as at the theatre. Now she feels the need to change the style of narration. She would like to express herself as if in a personal diary.

In the same period Carla says explicitly: 'I've decided to have my ears pierced.' My thoughts flash back to Carla's narcissism, to the difficulty she had in listening to my words, and to the problem of sexual indifferentiation (to the times when she would say: 'At my house we say front bottom and back bottom'; and when in our relationship we, too, were 'the front bottom and the back one' in a sterile coupling). Then I think of how she now reveals to me a marked differentiation towards femininity and a receptive capacity which she had always experienced as persecutory. I think of how she was closed to any sort of interpretation and of the turning point marked by her telling me that she was opening up her ears to my words and to her own feelings.

In reply I decide to communicate to her, by means of the intonation and warmth of my voice, my appreciation of her communication, saying simply: 'So now you can finally wear lots of nice earrings.'

'Yes,' she answers, 'as long as they're gold, because otherwise I'd get swollen ears' [i.e. the mumps].

As I pronounce the words 'earrings', I think of the acquired capacity to attach my words to her ears and of the recognition of an internal space inside her.

The patient as best colleague and the monitoring function

There are sessions which in terms of content may remain unexplainable. We may, however, furnish them with meaning by considering the patient's communications as unconscious descriptions of how the emotional movements of the last session can be observed and described. This description may use images from a vertex hidden from us, in the midst of the ongoing 'chorus' of indications about what is happening in the present session as it progresses.

Andreina begins the session by talking about a traffic jam that delayed her arrival. She goes on to speak about persecutions that she suffered because she had to do homework for some of her classmates. Then she asks if she can make a slight change in the appointment timetable.

This is an accurate description of the emotional overcrowding which had caused me to block the flow of transformation and, perhaps, resulted in inadequate interpretations, forcing her to increase her workload. It is also a way of sounding out my willingness to change, by asking for a slight shift in timetable.

With Marina the characters of the session change markedly, according to our mental functioning and my metabolic capacities. These characters range from 'the aunt who makes a good Sicilian-style sauce, cooking it slowly and adding sugar', to the same aunt 'patiently picking blackberries one by one to make jam', and to the friend 'who pretends, though she doesn't like him at all, to appreciate Kandinsky' ('canned din' = pre-recorded sound = the analyst's automatic functioning?). She goes on to introduce 'the hippopotamus that looked sluggish, but perhaps was dangerous', 'the violent classmate who threatens to profane tombs' (at a time when I was attempting to force open her silence), 'the one-way mirror they installed at school', and 'mother who is always respectful of the locked diary, reading only a few pages when her daughter *explicitly gives her the key*'.

And then there is Laura. Laura is particularly able to describe, in immediately comprehensible terms, what is going on in the session, as she sees it. If I am a moment late opening the door, she begins the session saying: 'When I come home, Sara doesn't come to the door right away. First she has to finish playing.' If I comment on what she says with sounds of assent, she says: 'There is a girl in my class who understands everything, but she never talks. She expresses herself in mumbled words that seem to be just noises.' If I am late, compared with what she expected, in answering she replies quickly: 'Sara was sleeping today. I let her sleep. That way when she wakes up she'll be ready to play, because she'll be rested.' If I am slow to pick up on her emotional state, she scolds me: 'The director was angry with the secretary because she made a lady wait in the waiting room even though she had an important appointment.' And if I beat around the bush or sidetrack, not receiving her emotions and not being fully permeable to her projective identifications, I hear: 'The teacher didn't come today. He probably went to play tennis, as he sometimes does.'

Needless to say, it would be pointless giving explicit interpretations of these 'signal lamps' of the functioning of the couple that light up from time to time, in contrast to what Langs (1975, 1978) and, occasionally, Rosenfeld (1987) suggest. This would mean breaking into or, even worse, 'profaning' the 'diary'. Instead we should constantly hold on to these signals in order to adjust the flavours of the interpretive cuisine, which must be regulated in such a way that the food, i.e. the feelings, can be 'touched', as Molinari Negrini (1991) has put it. In short, the couple is constantly narrating itself and its functioning.

Marcella tells me about two people leaving each other with considerable difficulty, adding that the question doesn't really interest her very much. And I ask: 'Are we sure? We've got holidays.' She immediately goes on to tell me about a little boy whose parents want to withdraw him from school because he feels mistreated by the teacher, and that he was very disappointed by the attitude of the school counsellor. It would be useless to express the patient's meaning in explicit terms, because it is not yet touchable. One must still approach it with 'pan holders', that is, with a certain careful detachment.

In order to document the journey which has brought me to my current position, I will present extracts from variously dated sessions, which illustrate different working models and their transformation over time. The destination of this journey is the notion of the field, as I conceive it today, exemplified in the final illustration, that of the 'little bison'. Here we will find, as Lussana (1991) points out, a shift in interpretive activity from 'raising unconscious phantasies to consciousness' to 'helping to receive, contain and digest emotional experience'.

Towards learning from experience

Interpretation or transformation?

Alessandro's asthma and his need for attention

Here are several sequences from a session which took place a few years ago with a seven-year-old boy named Alessandro. I will not go into the kind of problem we were facing, as my sole intent is to use the notes taken at the time to reflect on how the 'analytic dialogue' proceeded.

In the sequence of drawings we find the progressive formation of a container (see Figure 5.3). This is preceded by two pictures, drawn during the part of the session I have not reproduced, depicting a storm (Figure 5.1) and the arrival of Noah's Ark (Figure 5.2), the possibility of refuge.

The patient's verbal text

As soon as he comes in, Alessandro goes to the toy box, takes out the lion and the elephant, and has them 'play' together, saying that they are happy to see each other again.

At this point Alessandro takes the elephant and has it spray water at the thirsty lion. In rapid succession he takes the cow and the horse and has them walk together: 'They're going into the woods to eat.'

The analyst's working-through and interpretations

I focus on the most superficial, textual level of the communication and avoid interpreting a possible meaning of the choice of animals or their ferociousness. I say: 'Just like two friends getting back together.' I feel authorized to say 'friends', because in Alessandro's text the elephant and the lion 'play'.

I think that my phrase 'two friends' relieved him, just as the water relieved the thirsty lion. I also think that there has been a transformation from something potentially dangerous to something more domesticated (cow and horse). I'm keeping in mind the persecutory anxieties that thirst and hunger had activated in the horse and cow at the end of the preceding session, which had become the lion and elephant of the beginning of this session.

'This is what you hope we can do together.'

I am wondering whether it will be possible for me to take on the increase in work Alessandro is requesting: for some time now he has been asking me to increase the sessions to four.

Figure 5.1

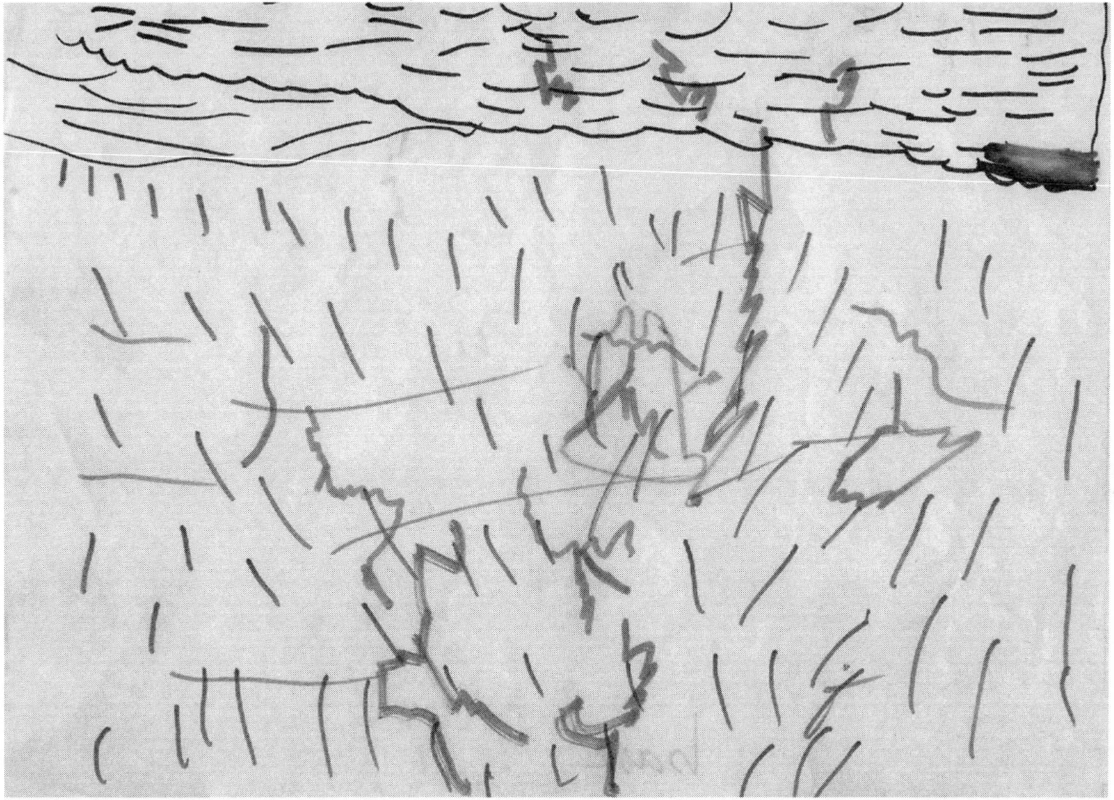

Figure 5.2

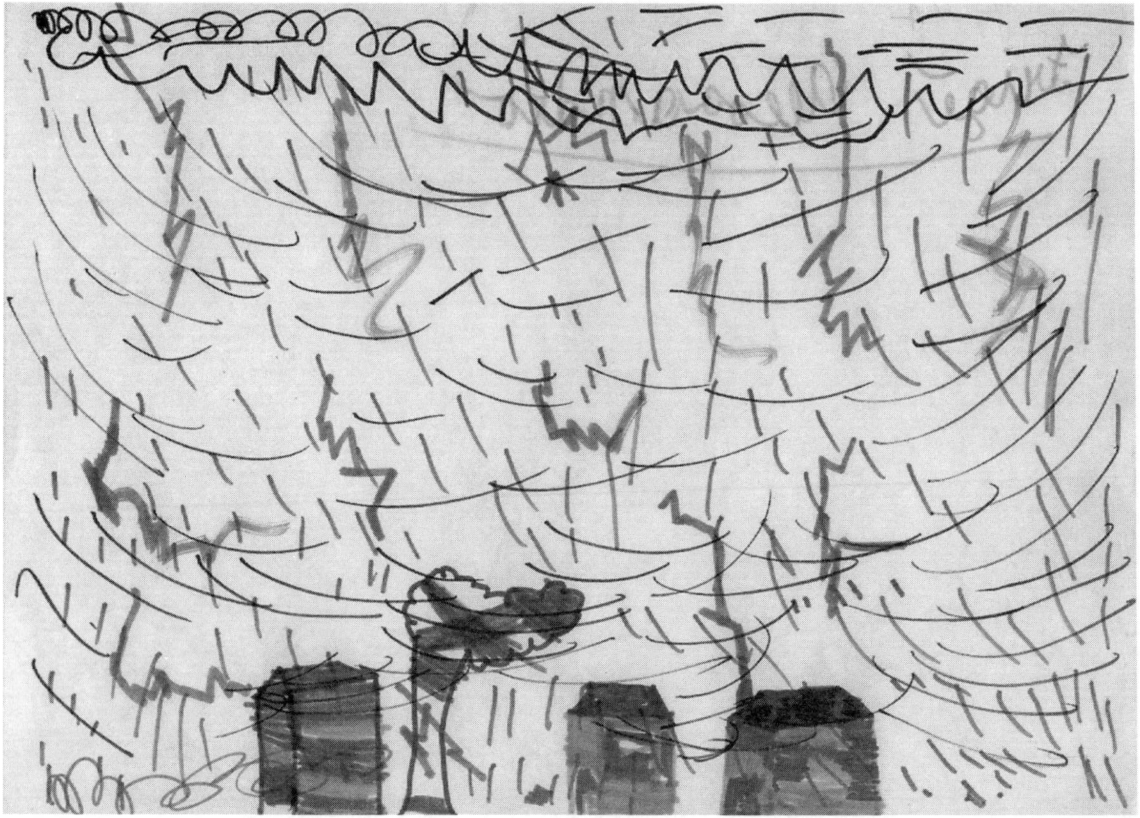

Figure 5.3

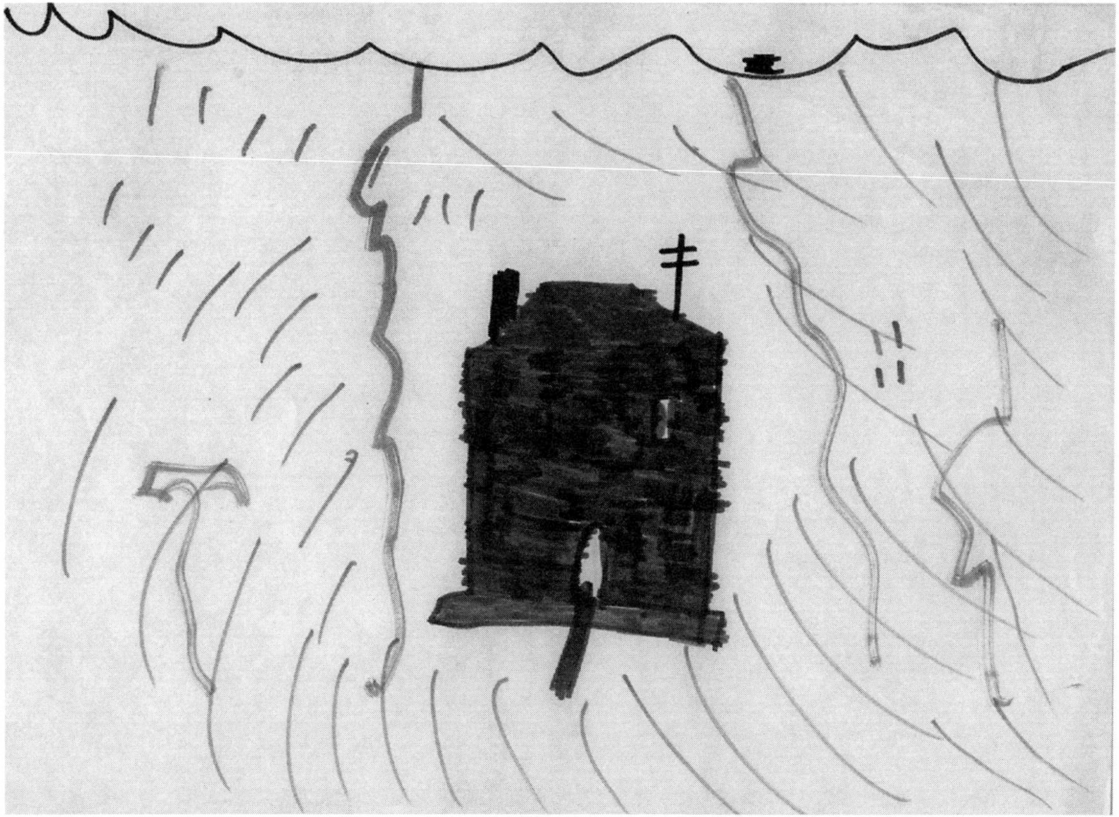

He takes the animals and puts them around a trough. A woman gives them feed. He sets a small horse aside.

I say 'Maybe you are afraid that there isn't enough room for the small horse next to the others.' I think it may have been premature to put into words what was perhaps my own preoccupation, that is, how to respond to his pawing (the horse?) demands (greed? the lion?). He may have been willing to wait, to set his pawing hurry aside, and to give me time. He recognized that the woman fed all the animals, or almost all; only the small horse was not fed immediately.

Yes, there's room for him, too. He takes the horse and has the dog carry him on its back: he has asthma and he has to be helped.

I think he is anxious because of my fear that I cannot satisfy his request (my 'you hope'), and because I interpreted the fear of exclusion and not his certainty that we were there working together, not pressured by haste.

He moves away from the window.

I understand that he feels oppressed. He moves away and tries to 'see', to find a view that can pull him out of his anxiety. I ask myself if I made him anxious when I said 'you hope' and 'fear that there is no room'. Perhaps I took the wind out of his sails, while he was trusting that we would work together.

He comes back toward me and says that he wants to draw. He takes some paper.

For a moment I am distracted, thinking about how to make space for him. In the emotional text there is now an urgency that penetrates me by means of projective identifications.

Alessandro drops all the sheets of paper: 'I don't know how to draw anymore!'

I am totally present again. I say 'Maybe you were worried because you saw I was distracted, and you were afraid that I wasn't interested in your drawing or in increasing the number of sessions.' I feel that I can now put into words what was in the emotional text but not yet in the explicit one.

He picks up the paper and asks me if I can put some sheets under his as a support so that he can draw better.

I do not say expressly that his request for other sheets of paper is a way of asking for more attention and openness toward his drawings and projects, including those concerning that session. However, I intensify my attention toward his communications.

[Subsequent passages, in which we work satisfactorily on the problem in hand are omitted.]

He draws a house, a clear sky, an aerial on the house, a chimney, and a window.	I think he is pleased with what I said and that he is signalling to me that we are in contact (the aerial) and close to one another (the affective chimney), and that we can see and understand (the window). I tell him that I think we understand each other and have a place where we can talk together. I say that the session is almost over and that we will continue next time.
He adds a storm to the drawing.	I say that my words may have destroyed the calm we had just established. I avoid giving expression to the anxiety of separation so as not to add another gale to the emotional turbulence.

Observations

This extract illustrates clearly enough, I think, the countertransferential labour, the working through of the patient's communications and the experiences activated, and at the same time the conviction that a solid relational axis is useful. There is still a strong tendency to 'give' an interpretation of what is happening. Although the interpretation is measured and not always expressed, it can still be regarded as the vehicle for a truth. The notion of the 'unsaturated' interpretation is not yet fully applied; more importantly, nor is it fully recognized that the patient and analyst can open up a path to thinking about something together which is totally unknown to the couple.

Also missing is the awareness of a jointly structured emotional field. I do not see my 'you hope' as an indicator of a $-K$ (Bion 1962) already circulating in the room when I distanced myself mentally. I was thinking about the increase in the number of sessions rather than about what was really being asked of me in the here and now: the increase of thought and capacity to think. I was not sufficiently attentive to the search for food in the woods and my withdrawal from the intimacy of eating together. (This withdrawal, moreover, should not be understood as reflecting feelings of guilt but rather as my taking on the burden of the couple's resistances, i.e. the shared −K.)

Basically, I do not even grasp what is happening when Alessandro puts the small horse aside (my 'you hope') so that the −K does not ruin the intimate relationship of mental exchange.

But if my need of perfection (my need in the field) cannot tolerate the exclusion of that 'you hope', then something is going wrong; or to put it another way, the small horse should not be saturated either as 'hurry' nor as 'you hope'. It should stay there until we see what narrative developments the story may reveal. The same holds for the asthma and the cow. In short, I still had in mind a rather saturating model, which, nonetheless, permits emotions to move about and dissolve. The transformation in the session is from the elephant to the lion, to the inhabited house, to the storm, in other words from the more primitive to the more domestic. But an opportunity for creativity has been missed. Instead of following an ordinary line, we might have followed sudden sparks of inspiration and produced more creative meanings together, as occurs in the final illustration I will present.

An unfortunate session: Luciano

Here follows a brief sequence from a session in which persecution is aggravated by the analyst's continuous, pushy activity of interpretation. He is inattentive to the young patient's capacity to receive interpretations; indeed, the interpretations become a further source of anxiety for the child.

Six-year-old Luciano arrives at our first meeting and takes some animals out of the toy box: the lion and the tiger, fighting in the jungle.

Analyst: They seem to be very angry.
Patient: Yes, very. Because they gave them bad food.
Analyst: Perhaps coming here today, to someone you don't know, and not knowing what to expect, is bad food.
Patient: The bull saw the lion's red tongue and became furious.
Analyst: Maybe it's when I talk to you that you get angry because you see my tongue.
Patient: King Kong is angry because they gave him bad food.
Analyst: Perhaps what I just said to you made you even angrier.
Luciano: (*Throws all the animals on the ground. Then he falls down, too. He adds:*) 'It was the wind.'
Analyst: The things I said to you seem to have frightened you a lot.

129

Observations

A situation is created in which there is absolutely no communication. The child indicates from the very beginning that he has been given 'bad food', an inadequate, saturating and unambiguous answer. But the analyst, more interested in deciphering meanings than in creating them together with the patient, seems to take on the child's fright and defend himself. His interpretations are mechanical, inappropriate, and they cause a negative transformation in the field, one of anger which rises until it reaches King Kong. At this point there is no longer a container for the rage, and the child becomes discouraged.

In another publication Bezoari and I (1989) quoted Marguerite Duras' *Pain*, in which she describes the feeding of a man who has survived a concentration camp. She explains that this feeding must be absolutely minimal, and that even then it will have catastrophic effects. That is to say, before introducing interpretations, we must ask ourselves whether there is *space* for them, and whether it is necessary to create this space together with the patient so as to make possible the progressive introjection of a *satisfactory relational modality*.

I cannot but return to what I said about the 'images' of the session, as providing feedback and a visual expression of what is happening in the emotional plot of the couple. The following examples illustrate this.

The turtle's shell

Carla is 8 years old. Following a session in which I was overly active in exposing some of her more sensitive aspects, linked to her more authentic part, she says that she saw a cartoon on TV in which Annette's mother communicated the wonderful news that Annette was going to have a little brother. But the mother died shortly after giving birth, leaving Annette not only an orphan but also with the burden of her newborn brother (as if to say that an excessively active and premature interpretation did, in fact, produce the birth and the experience of something new, but the separation was even more painful). Then Carla remembers another cartoon in which some turtles defend themselves from enemies who want to destroy them, and here she tells me about how she must equip herself with the shell of her defences in order to survive the pain of separation and the burden of new awareness (Annette's baby brother).

How much 'light' is tolerable: the observation of Andrea's answer

Returning to what was said about the novel by Duras, the following clinical sequence shows how an excess of 'truths' about the patient can generate persecutory feelings when such truths arise not from affective unison but from an attempt to arrive at our truths about the patient and inject them. This is confirmed by the images that are generated in the field and not perceived as indications of necessary defences which must be respected.

I will draw on three sequences which progressively show how much tolerability there can be to 'direct' interpretations, though I now believe that they could be largely replaced by the joint construction of shared meaning (Bezoari and Ferro 1990).

Andrea began analysis two years ago. He had difficulties in relating, especially at school, eating problems, and an emotional situation linked in part to a serious malformation of the skeleton. After a session in which I had proposed some interpretations which even I thought were violent, Andrea does a drawing which depicts Italy as a leg kicking a ball, Sicily. Tunisia appears as a fallen player shouting 'Foul!', while Sardinia is the torso and Corsica the head of a player who, with the addition of arms and legs, becomes a goalkeeper.

Andrea adds to the drawing: Italy is the analyst who gives interpretations, the fallen player is Andrea protesting, the ball is Andrea's head, and the save is made by a French goalkeeper.

In another session Andrea tells me about the hands of the Mona Lisa, which he saw on the front cover of a magazine. Then about Donald Duck. After that he makes a bird with building blocks: a duck.

I talk to him about the problem of hands, webbed hands and Donald Duck's bad luck. I speak about the fear that, in order to feel accepted, he has to make people forget that he is malformed by using his hands with extraordinary dexterity ('the teacher didn't notice for a long time because I used them so well').

He nods in agreement and then speaks to me about the mosquitoes that bite him, making little crusts ['croste' = scabs] form. From this I understand that I did not go too far with my interpretations, and they were not too persecutory (as they often are for Andrea when they touch on his malformation). And although the mosquitoes bite and cause some irritation, the crusts ['crostino' = toast] are also good to eat.

Here is the third sequence with Andrea. He comes to the session wearing his school overalls. This is the first time. I look at him tenderly. He says immediately: 'I can see the disappointment in your eyes.'

I interpret: 'You're afraid that if you arouse a feeling, it can only be one of disappointment, and that the little schoolboy cannot help but disappoint.'

He draws some extremely complicated levers. I say: 'It seems that the architect and scientist has replaced the boy.' He does a drawing depicting the head of a monster with sharp blades slicing an egg. This is how he perceived my interpretation. I was looking into him (without his collaboration) and making him feel as if he were being cut up into slices.

131

Observations

We still have the idea that an interpretation must be given in 'doses'. The problem is how the interpretation is felt by the patient, who is the only one in a position to signal this to us: kicking a ball, a crust, slicing an egg. Ultimately, there is still someone interpreting someone else's communication. We do not have the idea of an (emotional) text to develop together, as we will find years later when a child comes to the session with a chocolate egg with a surprise in it. He himself does not know what is in the egg, but the egg and the 'surprise' give birth to a session 'without memory and without desire', the entire meaning of which is constructed together.

An unfortunate sequence, or the time for understanding

Matteo is 10 years old. He is in his third year of analysis, and he has seriously malformed hands and feet, and great difficulty at school. To ensure that I am not just selecting examples to prove a point, I will present a sequence from some years ago chosen entirely at random.

At the beginning of the session Matteo tells me the story of a long film. The account is complicated and I get lost. I am also unable to find any interpretation that seems even vaguely appropriate. It is only by adopting a different listening mode that certain things recur and make sense in the patient's long story: 'vespa' [= wasp/type of motorbike], 'ape' [= bee/small three-wheel truck], the name of the main character, Mister Keller, which is sometimes pronounced 'Killer'. This makes it possible for me to interpret the persecution, in the transference as well, feelings of being stung, intruded into, threatened, chased, and struck by the killer analyst's interpretations, at least as regards a part of himself.

This takes us to the next session, in which Matteo talks about his cat and how it 'does its nails'. He brings in some drawings depicting his cat, one original (Figure 5.4), the other tracings showing the cat dressed in various ways (Figure 5.5). They all share the same feature, Matteo points out: the tip of the ears and of the tail are left off, as the picture 'overflows' the paper. His mother had told him several times to centre the drawing better, but 'for some reason I can't do it any other way'.

It is easy for me to point out to Matteo the connection between the cat's truncated ears and tail and the fact that he is missing the final phalanges – the 'malformations', Matteo calls them; the pawprint drawn in the first picture and Matteo's lack of fingerprints; the links between the malformations and the different guises in which the cat is shown (Figure 5.5). There is the cat as a Roman soldier, to which Matteo associates rage and fury; the supercat, with the power to perform extraordinary feats, such as flying; the

Figure 5.4

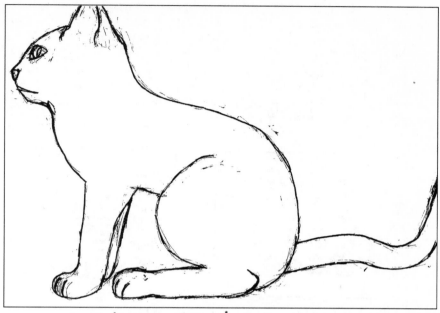

cat as president, an important person. Then there is the safecracker cat just escaped from prison, which represents the desire to understand everything at whatever cost; the policeman cat, i.e. the analyst; the Santa Claus cat representing birth; the newborn baby cat indicating Matteo's arrival in the world, like ET with malformations onto a planet inhabited by strange beings; and the Niki Lauda cat, with its mechanical engineering, accidents, and Niki Lauda's plastic surgery (Matteo has undergone plastic surgery several times). Considerable work is done on these associations in the course of the session.

In the following session Matteo shows me some very complicated drawings (Figure 5.6 (a), (b), (c)): combination locks, chains, bicycle locks.★ Nothing comes to my mind, so I wait, trying to understand.

I note that the combination locks have three cylinders (like the three sessions). Matteo explains that the locks do not work for various, extremely complicated reasons, which he explains. Then he picks up the book he brought and shows me airports and aeroplanes landing and taking off. Now

---

★Translator's note: All three drawings indicate joints which must be soldered (*Va saldato*). In Figure 5.6 (c) we have the following observation: 'This raised part serves to prevent the lock from being forced.'

Figure 5.5

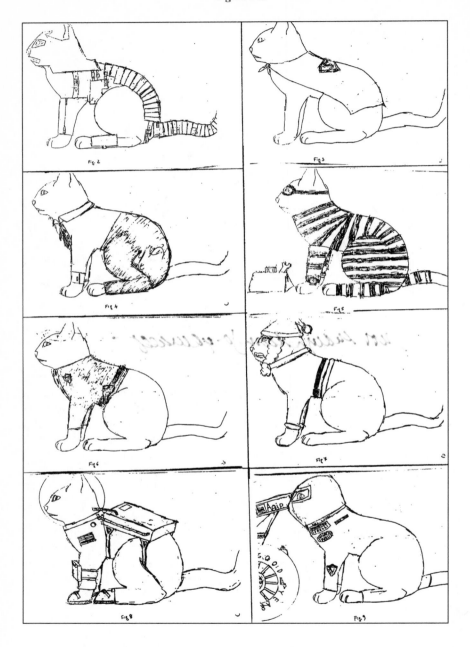

Figure 5.6a

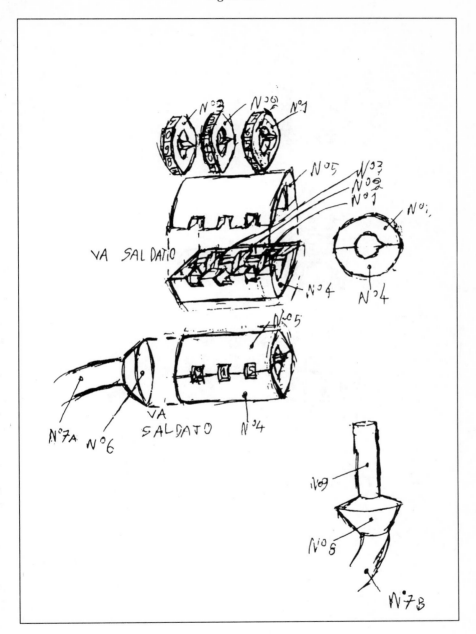

Figure 5.6b

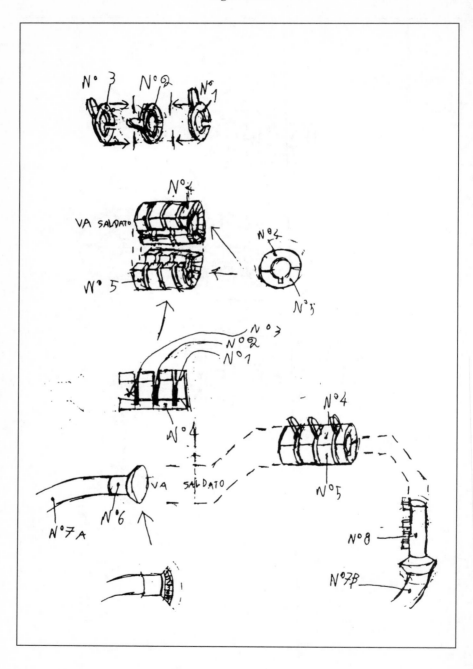

Figure 5.6c

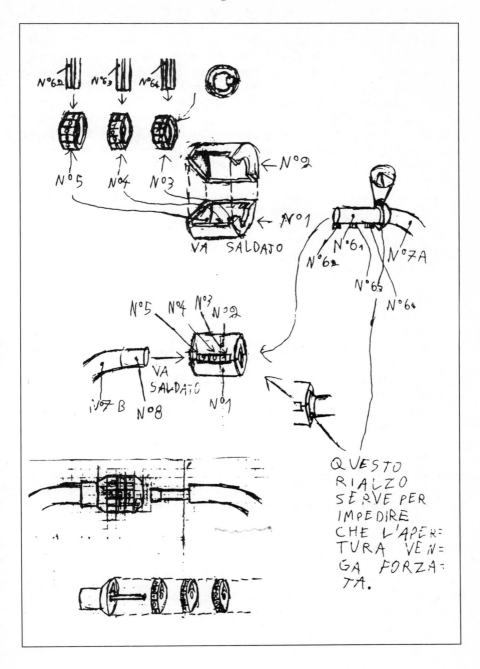

I think it is possible to draw connections. Matteo wants to hold me back, since today is the last session. He wants to lock me up in chains, but the locks and chains prove insufficient. Since he has difficulty expressing this desire in terms of suffering, he tries to give it a scientific guise. I do not find this interpretation satisfactory. It clarifies something to both of us, but it does not help us progress. The session proceeds with Matteo's promise to bring me the fortifications, castles and casemates he often draws. I have no associations to 'casematte' [casemates] = 'cose matte' [crazy things] = 'follia' [madness] = 'idea folle' [crazy idea].

In the following session Matteo brings a book with some sheets of paper in it. One falls out of the book and, reluctantly, he shows it to me: 'They're just cartoons. I traced two of them. The others I invented.' He shows me:

- A man sitting under a sign which says 'silence'. One of the wires from which the sign hangs breaks, and the sign falls on the man's head. The man is forced to disobey orders and shouts: 'Aahhh!'
- A person sitting in the waiting room of a doctor's office with hoards of bacteria specks falling off him. Another man comes in and says: 'I see your disease is frightfully contagious.'
- A man standing on a box with a rope around his neck, 'about to commit suicide'. A woman, his wife, comes in and says: 'Not today. I'd have to clean everything up, seeing that Mother is coming.'
- A football goal with four men in front of it: a coach, wearing a Scottish kilt, and three players. The coach says: 'Don't kick too hard. The goal cost a pound.'
- A man sitting in an armchair watching the TV. There is the accident in which Villeneuve jumps the race track. The man shouts: 'Blast!', but only because the car crashes through the back of the television, not because of any concern for Villeneuve.

Matteo himself tells me that he believes these cartoons may have some significance for the analysis, but he doesn't know what. I suggest he looks at them as a sequence, and he begins to advance some hypotheses. Together we construct a Matteo who has imposed silence on himself, as if with locks, who then breaks the silence when his suffering becomes very intense. Then there is a Matteo who is afraid he might have something that could cause others to avoid him. He is desperately afraid that whoever is near him may not perceive this desperation but rather direct his concerns and interests elsewhere. There is a Matteo persecuted by the interpretations/blows on the head which he receives in the course of the three weekly sessions. He is afraid of meeting his analyst, sitting in the armchair, who may not understand the drama of his accident (the malformations) and know how to be close to him.

At this point Matteo, nodding in agreement, opens up the book he brought from home. It is full of cars and shows lots of accidents. (I am quite concerned, knowing that he comes to the session alone by bike.) Then, I decide to tell him that I think he may feel so desperate sometimes, so angry and worried, especially afraid that no one understands him, that he may think it better to die, perhaps in an accident. He shows me a tow truck ambulance and then the dangerous phenomenon of aquaplaning, which occurs above a certain speed when the tyres of a car lose contact with the road surface. I suggest that what I said made him feel that I was close to him, but that he is also asking me to be very cautious when touching upon issues as painful as these. He is happy. He shows me a 'beautiful' drawing depicting a fortification; he says he will leave the drawings with me.

The session proceeds rather well. Matteo explains the drawing of the fortification in detail: an enormous enclosure wall, cannons and machine gun batteries on the roof, airplane hangars with planes, garages with jeeps, tanks, a heliport, runways, a great control tower. At this point I feel that I have moved away, taken up with the 'beauty of the material' and with thoughts of how to use the drawings. I seem to become like the man in the armchair, more concerned about his television than about the dramatic sequence that is unfolding before his eyes.

I provide a credible interpretation of the fortress in which Matteo has sought refuge to defend himself from the 'attacks' ('from the malformations understood as enemies', in Matteo's words), but I am distant from him and behaving like a geographer, a cartographer. Matteo's control towers and his tanks, like the safes of the preceding sessions, are able to launch an attack from within the fortress of the suffering boy. I am aware, however, that I am not giving interpretations that Matteo might feel as 'near'. He says that everything I said is true, but that I did all the talking. He picks up all the drawings he had intended to leave with me, rolls them up and takes them away, clearly disappointed. I am conscious of having acted out Matteo's fear: the person close to him is interested in the engineer, in the inventor, but not in the boy and in his suffering.

I will close with this bitter scene, reminiscent of the bitterness I felt at the end of the session. But the experience taught me not to write about Matteo immediately after the session. I was afraid that my interest in the material might prevail over interest in Matteo.

First comment: from a relational standpoint

The clinical sequence I have reported is quite long, but it seems to me that only in this way, reproducing detailed material from numerous sessions, is it possible to reveal the oscillation of the encounter between two minds and show how the mental functioning of the patient is not independent of the mental functioning of the analyst.

 When the analyst and the patient were on the same wave-length, the patient felt relieved, as in the interpretation of the comic strip sequence or when the patient commented on the interpretation of his desperation on the arrival of the tow truck. On other occasions, however, and especially when the analyst focused on the body (the malformations) and thereby retreated from encountering the patient's emotions, the patient withdrew and broke off contact.

The case of the locks is similar. Of course, many interpretations are possible, some that seem to come closer than others, but the most credible interpretation appears to be that which links the locks with the preceding session, with the fact that the analyst was unable to grasp the life in the first drawing of the cat. In fact, the interpretation centred on the malformations and not on the fact that there were parts (ears) that had not yet entered the session. One is reminded of Pinocchio who could scarcely be accused of not hearing, since Geppetto had not yet made his ears. The patient responds with a sequence in debased form that speaks about splits and about the limited scope of the analyst's vision (the ears and tail that remain outside the picture), but the analyst continues to propose legitimate, content-based interpretations. At this point the patient turns mechanical, and once again the analyst prefers contents, without understanding that it is the very lack of living interpretations that has caused the patient to become mechanical. Even in the sequence of cats the analyst does not realize how the emotion expressed in the first drawing (Figure 5.4), which he did not pick up on, becomes debased in the excessive clarity of the following drawings (Figure 5.5).

This lack of contact drives the patient in desperation to break the silence that he had imposed upon himself as a defence measure. Finally, the analyst manages to find the right wave-length again, though only for a brief sequence.

We could continue to examine the material in detail, but I think this can be left to the reader. Rather, I would like to propose some observations of another sort. Another way of reading the material, I would suggest, is as a spiral-shaped communicative process involving analyst and patient, a process in which the patient's answers are also comments on the analyst's interpretations, as described with considerable acumen by Nissim Momigliano (1984). The sequence can be considered either in the detail of each session or in the chain of several sessions. Thus the dream at the beginning of a session, for example, will probably be a comment on and an elaboration of the preceding session.

This way of seeing things requires us to pay special attention to an important point made by Langs (1984): the patient's material is contaminated and determined by the analyst's incomprehension. It is necessary then to be acutely aware of the current status of the relationship, since we find not only the patient's phantasies continually entering from the 'story' and from the 'inner world', but also comments and feedback which, if we are able to listen to them, can help modulate the work of interpreting.

It remains to be seen what makes it so difficult to establish a common wave-length. Here we must consider, I believe, what comes from the patient in terms of projective identifications, but also the natural oscillations of the analyst's mind, including the variations in the therapist's capacity to maintain contact with the split-off ('archaic' Bion would say) parts of his own mind.

Perhaps all this suggests that there is a mechanical way of interpreting which in turn mechanizes the patient. There is another mode – I would not know what to call it except 'living' – which originates there in the relationship and not in theories. This leads us to examine more deeply the oscillations between reverie, the capacity for interest in the other and the process of symbolization in the setting.

The capacity for symbolization cannot be understood, then, as a constant. Rather, it is a process involving many vicissitudes as it continually acquires and loses structure.

Perhaps it can be said that the only absence we analysts can know about is the absence that is revealed when we are in the session but the patient does not feel our presence. The patient may appeal to an internalization or to a helping object, or he may fall prey to panic or persecution, or, feeling alone and abandoned, become autistic (Matteo's locks). Then we could say that the symbolization of the absence is played out in the session (Di Chiara 1982).

It is also clear from the clinical material how often we, like the patient and together with the patient, feel the need for thermal shields. These may take the form of displacements in time and space of what is happening in the session, at least in the sense that all we can know about the analytic relationship is what is there with us at that moment, and nothing else (Nissim Momigliano 1981).

I would add one further observation about the activation of the analyst's reverie. The reverie may draw on something from the analyst's own experience or inner world, something that responds to and brings together possible meanings into one prevailing meaning provided, at that particular moment, with organizational capacity (Bion 1962; Gaburri 1982).

Second comment: from a field perspective

There is more to be said about the unfortunate sequence reported above. I understood very little of what was perceived as a persecutory way of entering the field. This attitude, once decoded and made clear, induced the patient to activate defence mechanisms (which represent a negative reflection of the way the analyst works). In other words, the patient multi-plies the objectives (the cats!) in order to facilitate his escape (while the ana-lyst multiplies his 'replicating' interpretations). Then he plugs his ears and, lizard-like, detaches his tail. Similarly, the analyst does not listen to or answer the feedback provided by the patient. The latter, faced with an excess of interpretations, 'does his nails', as yet undecided between anger and closure. In the same way, the cat 'defends itself' by becoming mechanical, just as the interpretations are mechanical. Then contact is once again established, and once again the fear of losing contact returns. The obtuseness of the inter-pretations about the malformations appears as a flight from the relationship and from asking oneself what was actually 'malformed', what was inadequate about the way the analyst entered the field, mechanized and without ears.

All this could be seen as the analyst's projective counteridentification as regards the patient's narcissism, but I find it more useful to consider it as a 'pathology of the field'. This pathology involves the patient's mode of functioning, in part mediated by the analyst's working mode, and requires the analyst to work through the problems of over-clarity (Meltzer 1976), narcissism, haste, fragility and persecution that emerge in the consulting room and in the relationship. At the same time, however, the analyst must respect the personifications and functional aggregates that 'live' in the room, as they are the concrete expression of the mental functioning of the couple.

Third comment: on the drawings

The interpretation of the drawings misses what is actually essential: the presence of a 'live' cat, as opposed to a cat made of blocks and drawn geometrically and without emotion, as it was months earlier (Figure 5.7). The situation recalls that of Poe's purloined letter. The multiplication of data obscures the 'felinity', the animality that enters the session and makes the relationship and the field itself dangerous – affects can kill – but are also terribly alive.

Time for transformations: Matteo's broom

The following is from another session with Matteo, when he was in his third year of analysis. I should recall that the analysis was requested because of episodes of incontinence alternating with intolerance of any sort of discipline and periods of rigid closure, with practically no contact with others. At the end of the first encounter I was told, almost by the way, that Matteo had serious malformations of the hands and feet. He had syndactylia

Figure 5.7

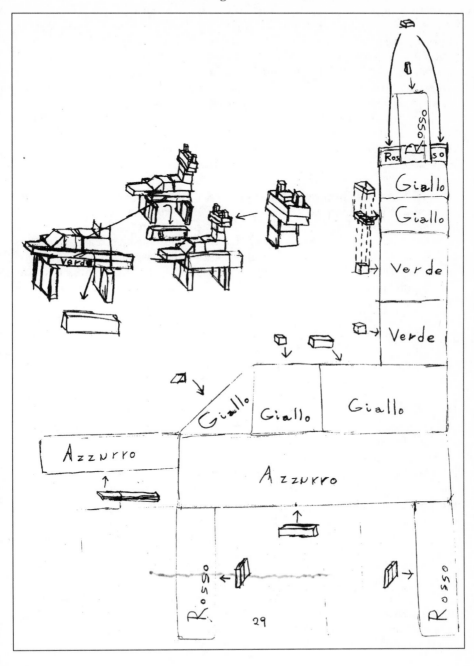

and was missing many phalanges, for which he had undergone surgery on numerous occasions, even from the age of a few months.

At the beginning of a session, after the third year of analysis, Matteo picks up an old drawing depicting the mechanical plan of a robot dog. Then he tells me he wrote a story for school. 'There is a family, with mother, father, two children and a dog, and they all go for a ride in the country. Suddenly a storm breaks out. Everybody runs back to the car, except the dog. The father gets out and goes to look for the dog. Just when he finds him, the broom falls from a scarecrow and frightens the dog, who runs away. After a while the dog meets a woman who wants to take him to a place where they take care of stray dogs. She is about to accompany him, when the dog again encounters the thing that persecutes him: a broom, with the bristles pointing upwards, that falls from a chimney sweep's bicycle. The terrorized dog runs away again. After some time he is picked up again, this time by another person. He is taken to a farm, where he is well taken care of. The dog stays there for a long time and develops an affection for his new owners. One day a car pulls up. It's relatives of the people who live on the farm, but the dog's former owners have come too. He leaves with them. On the way home, however, the girl realizes that the dog is unhappy. She opens the door and lets the dog out, so that he can run back to the farm.'

The story seems to me rich and full of phantasy. I have the impression, however, that the interpretation I provide is not equally 'beautiful', but rather flat and merely content-based. After the end of the session I understand why I had this sensation: it was an interpretation lacking in reverie. The thing that persecutes Matteo, the broom, had not reminded me of the second drawing Matteo had done in the analysis, about a year earlier (Figure 5.8). The drawing depicts a flower which, through associations, I had interpreted as hands whose fingers lacked the final phalanges. I have a sort of illumination.

At the next session Matteo is very distant. He speaks to me about very concrete things, like his days at school. Then he tells me about a song they are learning at school: 'La bella lavanderina' [The pretty washermaid], a song the washerwomen used to sing to while away the time.

I reflect on the sequence of the two sessions. I realize that it was the excess of anxiety, tied to the persecution of the broom, that obstructed the association 'broom = hand with truncated fingers', and that Matteo answered this absence of reverie by concretizing and moving away. My lack of reverie on 'broom = hand' corresponded to the way in which Matteo's parents and 'others' behaved with him. They blocked out the absence of phalanges, to which Matteo responds by almost hallucinating the fingernails, as he does when he relates in detail the 'clawing' of his cat. (Is this activating reverie on the part of Matteo?)

Figure 5.8

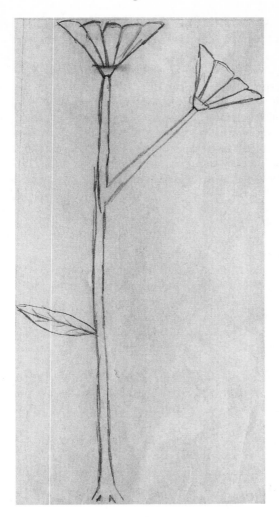

In the following session I decide to take a step back and propose all this to Matteo. I suggest that the 'Pretty washermaid' session was the patient's way of telling me 'we're not there'. When Matteo begins the session talking to me about mechanics I suggest that we step back and try to understand what happened, because he seems very distant to me: 'In the last session there was the pretty washermaid. Perhaps you were disappointed by my comment about your story. Maybe there's something I didn't understand.' I propose that we go back over it.

Somewhat thoughtful, Matteo summarizes the story. He adds that the broom appeared four times in the narrative. 'Well, I remember twice,' I say. 'I must have left something out.' He tells me that the third time was when the dog was taken to the farm. The unwitting farmer is sweeping the floor and the dog is terrorized. The man flings the broom out of the window so as to free both himself and the dog. The broom winds up in a tree. The dog in the meantime does the best he can. He rounds up the cows as he was taught to do by another dog. The fourth time comes near the end of the story, when the dog, let out by the girl, goes back to the farm. Just as he returns, the broom, which had been forgotten in the tree all this time, falls on top of him. The dog is frightened, but he sees the open door of the farmhouse and feels relieved.

The fact that Matteo adds these details already seems to indicate that it was a good idea to return to the story and that Matteo felt relieved to find me ready to provide refuge for him. Connecting the broom with something that makes him anxious, something he would rather forget but that keeps coming back, I say that his second drawing comes to mind. Without having to look in the folder of drawings he tells me from memory: 'Yes, I remember the flowers with the five petals' (Figure 5.8). I say: 'Yes, but also the hands and the feet: the four brooms that persecute the dog.'

Matteo is engrossed in thought. He confirms that this is something very difficult for him to think about, something he has always tried to free himself from. (The session continues.)

Let me add a marginal note here. After my first, flat interpretation Matteo had distanced himself. Now he can not only face the theme of persecution connected with his malformations, but also, towards the end of the session, allow other anxieties (autistic in nature) to emerge. He does this by telling the story of a film about the sinking of the *Poseidon*. For Matteo the story was like a long odyssey of passengers imprisoned inside a capsized ship (Matteo no longer the great megalomaniac painter but now the boy with and persecuted by malformations). The water is rising in the ship, and everyone is trying to escape through deadly dangerous metallic passageways and doorways. Finally the rescue team arrives and drills holes in the hull of the ship, saving the passengers, who were on the verge of suffocation.

Comment

Looking back, it seems to me that as I was too intent on immediately assigning a meaning, I did not allow time for transformations to take place through the elaboration of emotions rather than through the explanation of meanings, meanings which always appeared too exhaustive and cage-like, like the iron★ structure of the *Poseidon*.

I believe, on the other hand, that this is one of the limits of a theory based on the prevalence of the relationship, rather than on the idea of an 'unsaturated field', in which emotions and communications need considerable time to come together in often unforeseeable ways. I did not have enough 'ear' to recognize, for example, that it was the analyst's 'farm functioning' (♀) that gave relief to the dog, and that the dog felt persecuted by the 'brooms with the upward-pointing bristles'. The brooms, in fact, were the excessively active, almost phallic, interpretations, always ready to latch onto possible meanings and to return them menacingly, while the patient is left deprived of his most vital, living functioning.

I am rather satisfied with the reverie broom = hand with impaired phalanges, but only as a prelude to the understanding of a persecutory impact with excessively active interpretations (the almost electric bristles), interpretations that have not been sufficiently thought about (Manfredi Turillazzi 1978). In any case such interpretations are an expression of an activity carried out on the patient, or at least one from which he is excluded ('he is sweeping'), rather than with the patient .

Moreover, the need to assign 'roles' immediately to either of the couple prevented me from tolerating the presence of characters in the dialogue, characters understood as 'affective holograms' as yet to be thought about and developed in the narrative, a development dependent upon the interaction between the two minds and guided by the patient's signals and the analyst's working-through. All of this kept me from recognizing how wonderful was the entrance into the session of a dog as alive and intense as that of the story, an absolutely 'new' functioning for Matteo, who had long been just a mechanized boy.

Construction of a shared story: two authors in search of characters

This might be the place to cite positive illustrations showing how it is possible to 'narrate', to make transformations, to contain emotions that in time will be thought about and expressed. However, such examples have already been presented in the chapter on drawings – the 'little bison', 'the treasure', 'the aeroplane', 'Clarabella's nose' – so I will refer the reader to Chapter 2.

★Translator's note: 'iron' is the translation of the author's name 'Ferro' – he was being too cage-like for Matteo.

Theodore Lidz '50's
Luciana Di amant attachment + psychoanalytic language
Naidaur becomes anxious attachment

6

The child and the family group

secure vs anxious attachment

A child lives immersed in the emotional and affective culture of his or her family, and the family constitutes, in the full sense of the word, a group. Each family has its own emotional culture and its own way of organizing its defences against the anxieties it must continually face as a group (Gaddini 1976; Giannotti and De Astis 1989; Bonamino *et al.* 1992). Bleger (1966) gives us an incisive description of four different ways in which a family can organize its defences. A 'healthy' family functioning is one that is capable of organizing multiple and elastic defences. The others, in contrast, erect inter-locked symbiotic defences, schizoid defences, psychopathic defences and hypochondriac defences.

The *interlocked* group 'functions as a whole whose parts [not persons!] operate in a reciprocal interplay of relations and interdependent compensations'. There is an indiscriminate narcissistic structure which never realizes a differentiated personification.

At the other end we find the *schizoid group*, in which each member *disengaged* 'embodies the indiscriminate group as an internal object and creates a symbiosis with that group inside itself. In reaction the group blocks emotional relationships within itself, and the relationships become cold and distant.' In both types, defences are inadequate to protect the groups from fusion and loss of identity, because, lacking differentiation, they are unable to evolve.

Midway between these two lie the psychopathic and hypochondriac family groups. In the former there is 'a flight of an interlocked group from claustrophobic fusion'. In the latter, hypochondriasis or psychosomatic phenomena are equivalent to psychopathy.

Bleger stresses that normality depends on these defences being mobile and that it is normal for such defences to emerge whenever there is change, whether inside or outside the group. He also notes that 'the family group is the repository of the most immature and symbiotic part of the personality' and that it tends towards stereotyping to keep the psychotic part under control so that 'the more discriminate and adapted part of the personality can develop outside the group'. *narcissism - denial of need*

Bleger also points out that it is useless simply to observe the family group. What is needed is an 'operative investigation', that is, one in which we advance hypotheses, introducing them as new variables in family group dynamics. These hypotheses are then confirmed or corrected by the answers we receive to these suggestions and are then reformulated. So the observer is not neutral but participates in and interacts with the group.

Another quite accurate description of the family group appears in a highly concentrated little volume by Meltzer and Harris (1983). The authors examine and describe various types of family structure and discuss the consequences on the upbringing of children. They identify seven main ways of learning that are transmitted within the family.

1 *Learning from experience.* This is possible when the individual participates in an emotional experience that can bring about a change in the structure of his/her personality and that enables him/her to learn ways of thinking about how to solve a problem.

2 *Projective identification.* Although the desire to acquire the object's qualities immediately is limiting, it is possible through projective identification to gain access, if to a lesser extent than is often supposed, to the capacities and knowledge of the other. There is, however, always a risk of slipping towards feelings of omniscience and superiority.

3 *Adhesive identification.* In situations in which the object is not emotionally available, the only alternative is to 'hold yourself together' in other ways, as in the phantasy of sticking to the surface of external objects. The individual inevitably acquires capacities to learn social roles, but not their corresponding functions. *narcissistic mother*

4 *Learning by 'scavenging'.* This way of learning is based on the idea of theft and is typical of the envious part of the personality. What is 'stolen' cannot be used freely, because it carries with it the guilt of the theft itself. Consequently, secrecy and inhibitions are its corollaries.

5 *Obsessive collecting.* This way of learning is characterized by the omnipotent desire to control objects, depriving them of their freedom, force and vitality.

6 *Delusional learning.* Here only what is hidden counts. The nuances and details of appearances conceal the ultimate truth.

7 *Superficial learning and subjection to a persecutor.* This involves a tyrannical method which imposes mechanical learning.

Meltzer and Harris (1983) go on to distinguish various types of possible communities, such as the benevolent community of the combined object, the supportive maternal community, the supportive paternal community, the parasitic maternal community, the parasitic paternal community and the paranoid community. Then they describe the 'family organization' at the level of basic assumptions, the emotional roles and functions of the family (to generate love, arouse hate, promote hope, sow desperation, contain depressive suffering, transmit persecutory anxiety, create confusion, think). Finally they distinguish five types of family on the basis of these functions.

1   The *'couple family'*. In this type the introjective functions of the couple are not divided into masculine and feminine but rather lie within a spectrum in which, at one end, the mother tolerates the impact of the children's projective identifications and, at the other, the father 'imposes a limit on the evacuation of mental waste'. The vulnerability of this structure lies in the fact that each member is irreplaceable in the maintenance of a proper balance.

2   The *'matriarchal family'*. In this situation discipline is maintained by appealing to feelings of guilt.

3   The *'patriarchal family'*. Here discipline is severe and the children are subjected, leading to their rebellion.

4   The *'gang family'*. This structure is quite narcissistic and emphasizes seductiveness and permissiveness.

5   The *'reversed family'*. There is no introjective function and there is a drive toward unrestrained actions.

The authors continue with a description of the mental states of the individual (the adult state of mind, infantile bisexual state, masculine or feminine infantile states of mind, girl–gang or boy–gang states, inverted or perverted state of mind). I can only recommend this extremely valuable work as essential reading. Indeed, it is so dense that no summary but only direct study can do it justice.

Children are quite permeable to the projective identifications of the family group. Indeed, I would not hesitate to say that the child is nearly always the 'carrier' of the often dormant illness of the entire family group. Children adopt the unconscious functioning of the group and take on its specific anxiety. This is not very different from Pichon-Riviere's (1971) position when he says that the prognosis and diagnosis for each patient must take the family group into consideration: the diagnosis because the patient is the 'depository' of the family illness, and the prognosis because his reinsertion depends partly on the group's capacity to take back some of the anxiety deposited in the patient. If this is true of all patients, it is especially true of children, who in the course of therapy must not only deal with their own internal group but also continue to be immersed in that, often pathogenic, milieu which is the basic emotional culture of families. Although this culture may undergo change, through the transformations that the therapy brings about in the child, it will also need help to be transformed if the child is to make further progressive, evolutionary changes.

The family's 'illness' is generally latent and emerges thanks to the symptom (or symptomatology) of its most exposed and healthy member. In the more fortunate cases, the symptom may signal a family dysfunction in the management of group anxieties, thus making it possible to reorganize the defences against such anxieties or, if they are too intense, to re-elaborate them.

What we have just said has important consequences. It follows that it is *necessary*, especially in the case of younger children, for another therapist to take charge of the parents to ensure that the necessary readjustments are made. The meetings may even be occasional. After all, it is the child's therapy that functions as the instrument of change, though it must not be forgotten that the child continues to live in the environment which brought about his or her illness and that it is essential to transform this environment.

The other consequence is that it is useful to have a preliminary meeting with the parents or, if the therapist is experienced enough, with the entire family group, in order to foster an understanding of the relationship between the family culture and the pathology of the child. If someone were available to take charge of the family, as Meltzer (1964) suggests, it would be possible to see the child directly without knowing anything about him. This approach is possible, however, only if the therapist has adequate expertise and if she or he can be sure that someone else will see to the family (Lussana 1989).

More commonly, the analyst meets the parents and does not find it difficult to gather useful information. This first encounter can be listened to and 'relived' in various ways. The therapist gathers information about the child, about the functioning of the parents as a couple, about the anxieties connected to the problem at hand, about the family's group dynamics. I would like to draw attention, however, to a particular listening vertex, one that considers the encounter as though it were a group session in which what counts is not the single communication of each participant but rather the whole of the communications seen as the product of a unitary 'group mind'. This overall product can be divided into various parts or functionings: the father character, the mother, the child, and whatever other characters are mentioned. Let me try and illustrate what I mean.

A family that 'sticks together' and the two photographs

When Maria's parents arrive for the consultation, they are quite alarmed. The father, a medical doctor, was afraid we might be dealing with psychosis.

I ask the parents to explain the problem. Maria's mother takes out two photographs. One shows Maria (whom she calls 'the girl') and the other Maria alongside 'her older sister'. Maria is 12 and her sister 19. I am immediately relieved by the mother's presentation. I think that she has understood and is unconsciously presenting the problem: the co-existence of a 'girl' and a 'young woman'. It is this cohabitation of two ways of being that has disoriented Maria and her parents.

Maria's performance at school is a bit weak but not so weak as to attract the attention of her teachers. During the summer Maria was worried about the load of *homework* she had to do, and this caused her some anxiety. Of course her real homework or task was to find harmony, to integrate her infantile and adult aspects.

At the end of the summer she sold some old things, but with the money she earned she wanted to buy a doll. Her mother was shocked and fought with her to make her change her mind, saying that now she was grown up, she'd have to get married, and have children. Maria spoke about suicide because of all the *homework*.

Her parents, overinvolved as they were in what was happening to their daughter, found it difficult to regulate their behaviour. They were frightened by Maria's need to regress and her demand that a place be recognized for the 'child'. They were even more alarmed by Maria's tears over the loss of a teacher. They were disoriented because, after she had received a compliment from a friend, Maria refused to put on a dress again that revealed her slender figure. At the same time they don't understand why their daughter is proud to wear modestly high-heeled shoes.

Finally, there is Maria's disorientation, coinciding with the first signs of puberty. She was terrorized at having found a 'hairy worm' in her bed and asked to sleep with her father. This request, on the one hand, led her to realize that she had Oedipal desires, and on the other, once granted, confirmed that she was still a child.

It was enough to meet the parents for a few months to help them find the right balance, to discover the meaning of what was happening and to recognize their own difficulty as middle-aged parents. As they accompanied Maria's growing up, they themselves were running into the problems of mid-life crisis.

Bianca Sibert and He-Man

I receive a telephone call: 'I want an appointment because my son *isn't going to the bathroom*, and he hardly ever goes.'

At the first meeting, as I receive the man I suppose to be the one who telephoned and the mother, I immediately think: '*They certainly are clean*', as I notice their orderly and immaculate appearance.

They tell me that Fabrizio, their son, is '*not jealous, not aggressive, and he shares his things* with other children . . . *he hugs them*'. The mother says: 'He never never wants to poo-poo . . . he wants to do it standing up, as if he were peeing . . . just like a boy.' She comments on her husband: 'Sometimes he is very worried and has guilt feelings, and then I wonder whether it's my *fault* because I insist that Fabrizio should eat.'

The husband: 'Maybe it's my wife's *fault* because sometimes she loses her patience . . . it's our *fault* because we're out of the house a lot . . . I let him watch "Bianca Sibert" on TV, but I don't let him watch "He-Man". But he's not afraid of the dark. He says, "Dad, let's look for the *crocodile* under the bed."'

They go on to talk to me about the nursery school, the family, the uncle who gave him a *rifle*. 'But I,' says the father, 'didn't want him to bring it home.' When Fabrizio is with a smaller child he says 'hee . . . hee . . . hee', and he fondles him. Of course, there are many images that are evoked by the contact with me. The most positive seems to be the desire to know and to go and find the 'crocodile' that they mentioned.

Let's set aside for the moment the more relational level and the interaction with me. (Of course I did speak cautiously a few times, to help the parents along in their narration and to address the fear of bringing negative aspects in contact with Fabrizio. I thus participated in the narrative development of the meeting.) I would like, rather, to make a sketch of their communications. If I were capable of rendering them graphically I would choose the colour, the emotional hue of my experience – '*They certainly are clean*' – and the images: 'child terrorized by poo-poo'; 'I let him watch "Bianca Sibert"'; 'I don't let him watch "He-Man"'; 'No rifle'.

These images seem to suggest a possible meaning and the creation of a story, as regards both the group functioning as one single mind, and, quite probably, as regards Fabrizio. It is very likely that the problem has to do with the guilt feelings concerning the primitive and violent parts/feelings/emotions (which are denied, cleaned up, cancelled – 'not jealous . . . not aggressive . . . not violent'). In connection with these parts there is the fear that they can be retained anally, that they cannot be worked through, thought about, transformed. There is a feeling of guilt about the primitive and violent parts, parts that have not been civilized. There is an attempt to propose as an antidote, artificially, a cold environment where there is room for Bianca Sibert and her pedagogic pseudo-environmentalism but not for He-Man and his primitive stories made up of splitting, strong feelings, love and hate, life and death, good and bad (Skeletor), the rifle, the poo-poo, the dirt. Probably also there are split-off parts not yet thought about and, returning from the group of individual minds, split-off parts of the father, the mother and, consequently, of the child. These products of splitting do not permit an approach, a working through; the more they are retained, the more frightening they are, and the more frightening they are, the more they are uncontainable. The only alternative is to *hold them back*, even though the child would prefer to face everything 'standing up', like a man.

The images chosen for my 'sketch' are also the most evocative in my reverie: *no He-Man*: They are able to pronounce only the first part of He-Man: 'hee ... hee', just like Fabrizio with smaller children, but the second part, 'man', the more active, primitive part, is lost.

Bianca Sibert: the North Pole seal, cooling off sentiments, metabolizing. We should not forget to add 'the uncle who performs a more paternal function', and the capacity to desire 'to go and see the crocodile', to go, that is, and look for and face the split-off parts that are still hidden and have not yet been thought about, the frightening parts.

Of course, the associations could continue, and find confirmation in the subsequent analysis of Fabrizio. His problem, in fact, was fear of his own emotional incontinence, regarding anger, aggressiveness and jealousy. During the analysis the *crocodile* gradually turned into a tiger, a lion and, finally, an affectionate little monkey that played with *coco*-nuts and the *man-drill*, as his father began to call his son when he made his first amorous conquests at nursery school.

Certain phrases that take shape in the encounter seem to come closer than others to the emotional truth of the mind, as though they contained evocations of images that may belong to ongoing daydreams, through the alpha function of dream-thoughts in waking life. It is as if certain images were, and rendered possible, the echo of 'dream-like flashes' that reach us, messages that arrive from the 'dream' of the minds of the group and that allow us to create a meaning through drawing, or, perhaps I should say, through the *dream* we may have of the encounter itself.

Clearly, I have intentionally ignored the relational level of the encounter, that is, the connection between the images evoked, the moment and the nature of my, albeit cautious, communications. Once therapy has begun, it is impossible to ignore this level, because what we can know about this situation is only what comes out in the interchange with the patient. And we ourselves contribute to structuring the images that are produced in the field. So I would consider the interpretation given above as merely an exercise on a possible, supposed text, which ignores the interrelation with my own contributions: and this, of course, is impossible.

When there is a twofold request: from desperation to the fertile encounter

I receive a request for consultation for 'a boy' from a person whose history is marked by a mixture of despairing events and actings out. As the person speaks, I also get a feeling of desperation. I don't know what to think of what

I am being told. Maybe I have to change my view of the idea that, as long as there is a request, an analysis can always be attempted. It seems, however, that it is increasingly unclear who needs help. I am beginning to think that the request concerns not merely the actual son but also the person who has called me.

The woman adds that she is not sure whether she should allow her husband to 'recognize' the child, and that she is afraid the child might grow to love the father and become disappointed; he is greedy, interested only in his wealth.

I decide to skip all the possible implications and transferential movements in the here and now and try to 'recognize' the girl part. I make an attempt to draw on characters from Mickey Mouse: Uncle Scrooge for the greed, Donald Duck for the mishaps, the basset hounds for the dreaded break-ins.

The patient (this is how I will refer to her now) is amazed for a moment. She says that she 'can't see well out of one eye' and that she will have to have an expensive eye operation. Sometimes she thinks that the man she married is not the unreliable cad she has always thought him to be. Once, she remembers, he took his son by the hand and showed him around the whole fertile farm, saying that if she allowed him to recognize the boy, it would all become his. There is no point in continuing. The recognition of the boy arouses great hope, and the interpretation based on Mickey Mouse reveals (*structures!*) a farm and fertility, things that suggest the possibility of an encounter, of work to be done. Moreover, the analyst is now able to recognize the desperation he sensed at the beginning. He is able to recognize that, in thinking he has to 'change his way of looking at things', he is successfully taking on the projective identifications arriving from the patient. What is more, even the 'story' narrated by the patient is saved. It is not subjected to lacerations or decoding. This is a story involving two minds and their encounter – it is a couple-specific story. True, it is transmitted through repetition, the outward projection of phantasies, but it is transmitted above all by projective identification. After all, what is of interest to us is the unknown story, the story that cannot be narrated directly through images, the story of psychic events so primitive, sometimes so catastrophic, that they are always set elsewhere. Hence the 'desperation' that gave rise to the reverie on Mickey Mouse. It was an answer to the desperation of a child considered dead and buried under actings out, and whose apparently atrophic strings resounded, once the child was given an answer evoked by the transmission of an emotion.

The twofold nature of the request was revealed and sorted out in subsequent meetings. The patient's son needed help, and therapy was necessary for him to be able to 'start up' again in the new situation that had taken shape. The patient herself also needed analysis. She was unable to forgive herself for the experiences which had ultimately made it possible for her to survive in

155

a family situation which got off to a truly tragic start, experiences from which she managed to rise up with dignity and strength.

This last example reveals a vertex which is quite different from that of Sibert, since it shows that the first meeting plays an important role in determining the structure of the future relationship.

Many other illustrations could be given, of course. It could be shown, for example, how the first meeting with parents can provide information about the whole range of the child's problems. But my aim was to point out the different possible levels and interpretive keys that can be used in the initial encounter, ranging from the more descriptive and 'external' to the field oriented, and from that in which the characters are considered as people, to that in which they are considered as internal characters, or as 'functional aggregates'.

A geography of the theoretical model in use

I would now like to draw a summary sketch of the theoretical model which I have developed and shown in use in the preceding chapters. The model results from what I feel to be a fruitful convergence of many concepts elaborated by Wilfred Bion and by William and Madeleine Baranger.

The basic idea is this: the patient and the analyst create a relational and emotional field (Baranger and Baranger 1969a, b; Baranger, Baranger and Mom 1983; Corrao 1986, 1988) within which pockets of resistance are formed which only the analyst's working-through can overcome. But quite often this is not enough, because the analyst's countertransference is unconscious, so he is unaware of much of his involvement in the relational field. If it is true, as Bion says (1983), that the patient 'always knows what is going on in the analyst's mind', then we can expect the patient to pick up on and describe the analyst's movements as he gets closer or moves away. It follows, then, that the creation of the characters of the session is a development of the countertransference by the patient – the analyst's 'best colleague' – who keeps on signalling what is happening in the field, but from vertices which are completely unknown to us. Our task is to make these vertices our own, so that the emotional forces which are present in and which indeed constitute the field may be worked through and undergo genuine transformation (Ferro 1991, 1996).

Of course, this is only one way of listening, and if it were the only one, we would be left with a relationship which pointlessly winds around itself. Instead, it is a vertex that *oscillates* in harmony with other approaches: the one which places more emphasis on the external 'historical' aspects of the patient's communication and that which pays more attention to his inner world of phantasy.

The decoding of meanings is replaced by the construction of new meanings. New 'stories' can be thought up by the analytic couple, stories which, once worked through and transformed, find their place back in the main 'story' (Barale 1990; Ferro 1991; Bezoari and Ferro 1992, 1996). The first thought I would offer at this point concerns the importance of the way in which projective identification, seen from a markedly relational point of view (Bion 1962, 1967b; Baranger and Baranger 1969c; Sponitz 1969; Ogden 1979, 1982; Manfredi Turillazzi 1985), makes possible a continuous exchange of emotional elements, which gradually find that they prefer to be expressed in words. Projective identifications express the specific and subterranean emotional state of affairs between the members of the couple who, through dreams, drawings and anecdotes, find a way of expressing and narrating what is going on in the depths of the relational exchange.

The interpretation is not something which, dictionary in hand, makes it possible to pinpoint a meaning (as is sometimes suggested by a Kleinian model with its repeated references to the unconscious phantasy of the patient). It is, rather, the proposal of a meaning, which is never exhaustive but always taking shape; 'unsaturated', as Bion puts it. This 'hypothesis' uses the couple's emotions as a springboard to arrive at new, more complex and clearly defined meanings which in turn transmit affects to both members of the couple (Bezoari and Ferro 1989, 1990, 1991c; Meltzer 1986a; Abadi 1987).

The characters of dialogues, drawings, games or dreams (it matters little through which door they enter the session) bear witness to the two minds' processing of the reciprocal projective identifications and make it possible to communicate, through images and shared stories, what is going on between the members of the couple. In this sense the characters are born through the relational text's need to express emotions and affects.

The interpretation, then, is a sort of 'duet', a product of the relationship which requires the participation of both minds, each in its own way (Bezoari and Ferro 1994). The analyst's intervention has highly unsaturated semantic potential, which leaves room for the active participation of the patient. This is what Bezoari and I meant (1989) when we spoke of 'weak interpretations' – adapting the philosophical notion of 'weak thoughts' (Vattimo 1983) – as opposed to 'strong interpretations', which are presented as exhaustive and which provoke closure.

The locus of asymmetry, the much emphasized dependence of the patient, is shifted in the analyst's working-through (Brenman Pick 1985) and in his/her continuous work. This work consists in receiving, transforming and 'labelling' the patient's projective identifications, modulating interpretations, listening to the way in which the analyst's observations are received (Langs 1978; Nissim Momigliano, 1984; Joseph 1985; Molinari Negrini 1985), paying attention to the characters that enter the session in the guise of the patient's responses, and accepting responsibility for what happens in the field, including the countertransference. In my view, the analyst 'depends' upon the patient's mental functioning and must supply him with elements of growth 'processed' in such a way that the patient can receive them. The patient, on the other hand, depends upon the analyst's capacity for reverie and working through.

It is the analyst's task to transform the patient's beta elements, to receive them, digest them, narrate them, and allow them to take on a symbolic form which, in Meltzer's view (1981a), is the birth of children in the shared analytic bridal bed. In addition, of course, the analyst must not bombard the patient with his own beta elements.

The approach to listening I am proposing entails a fully receptive role in monitoring the field. It pays total attention to the transformations of the figures of the analytic dialogue, making it possible, on the one hand, to view ourselves and the patient from the latter's vertex and, on the other, to avoid reducing all our operations to interpretations pertinent exclusively to the relationship or the transference. This allows us to make direct use of the *characters evoked* as pawns that can be moved around, while never forgetting their fully relational meaning (Ferro 1993c, 1994, 1998b).

What is more, we must take into account that the interpretation has to use the same level of communication as that used by the patient. This guarantees that all the semantic penumbra suggested by the patient will be received. This level of communication emerges from the awareness that the prerequisite for any symbolization is the alphabetization of the patient's beta–elements (Ferro *et al.* 1986b). Although the decoding of meaning may have (or may have had) significance for the neurotic parts of the personality, for the psychotic parts it is only a genuine operation of alphabetization which makes the transformation of beta-elements possible.

And it is, once again, the patient who continually expresses how much this process is occurring or is being avoided. The patient is constantly telling us what we are like for him, from vertices which remain entirely unknown to us. We must, however, perforce remain aware that 'his' problem may enter the field precisely thanks to a door which we ourselves open.

When we function with good availability and permeability, we are powerful receivers and often interpreters of the patient's projective identifi-cations. In any case the patient will eventually tell us, in one way or another, how we are receiving or not receiving such projective identifications.

The characters that communicate or express this may, in turn, be 'written in' from different worlds: from childhood memories, current events in the patients' lives, dreams, phantasies and so forth.

Suppose, for example, that after a session which I consider to have been fruitful, the patient dreams he goes into a field where his father has four cherry trees, and that he finds many people there, all of whom are really his friends but who have already picked the fruit. Suppose this same patient goes on to say that in his dream he is disappointed, not so much because there are no cherries left for him but because he is thus deprived of the pleasure of taking them to his classmates. In such a case, I sense that the patient is signalling to me that I am overdoing it with my interpretations, that I am taking away from him the pleasure of participating in the picking, in the labour, and, above all, in the sharing (Winnicott 1971b). These are the feelings I must get in touch with: the pleasure of 'being the one to bring presents to his friends', the 'disappointment' and so on, although this means giving up further interpretations which would leave all the cherry picking to me.

I should stress once again that this approach to listening cannot remain isolated, because if it is isolated it results in a relationship which revolves around itself. On the contrary, we must strive to achieve a continuous oscillation of listening vertices which take into account the past, the internal world, the phantasies and the relationship. It is the last of these which I consider to be foremost and endowed with greatest psychoanalytic depth. This vertex, I repeat, concerns what the patient says (or does not say) as a running narrative commentary on what is going on between the two minds in the session, a perspective which we must share if we are to reach the patient.

The analyst, like the student of characters in literary narratives, must find his bearings in the midst of 'a hierarchy of codes working at the same time' (Hamon 1972).

Another oscillation I would like to draw attention to is that between wide-angle and close-up views, a sort of play of different lights that may at times illuminate the entire field and thus show the movements deriving from the couple's internal groupings and the 'characters of the session' as they enter the scene, move about, appear, exit and change. On other occasions the light may focus on one of the couples or relationships in the field which, at that particular moment, the analyst feels to be the most significant. In this case there ensues an interruption and a transformation of the relational phenomena of the field, which will then regroup in a different way.

The 'strong' effect of the transformation of the field is described very suggestively in a short story by W. Allen, 'The Kugelmass Episode'. A twentieth-century man living in New York manages to 'enter' *Madame Bovary*, with the help of a magician, and a love affair develops with the heroine. The consequences are extraordinary for Flaubert's novel, since the critics are suddenly faced with a new character and new events which wreak havoc on the codified text, but also for the everyday life of Mr Kugelmass, who finds Madame Bovary entering his life when she asks him to take her to New York. It is only through the decisive intervention of the magician that Kugelmass and Bovary are allowed to return to their respective worlds and stories.

Another example of the different levels which may exist between the characters' dialogue, the narrative text and possible new stories and plots is to be found in Diderot's *Jacques le fataliste et son maître*. Here the dialogue between the two main characters is repeatedly interrupted by the interference of external events, by the need to pay constant attention to where their horses are taking them, but above all by the intrusions of the author who, at the appearance of each new character, remarks on all the potential plots and stories that could be told.

Getting back to our point, then, the stories told by the couple through the characters make it possible to transform the underlying emotions and to open new paths of meaning (rather than to decode meaning). The session is comparable to a countertransference dream, as it allows the analyst to regulate his mental and interpretive state (Barale and Ferro 1987, 1992) in the search for the specific functions which the patient needs. Thus, following a somewhat doctrinaire interpretation in the transference, Maria tells me about her grandmother who made her 'wear a tight corset'. In other words, if an interpretation simply decodes, it ends up by imprisoning communication and imposing one meaning to the exclusion of all others.

On the other hand, the unsaturated joint construction of meaning is a guarantee of fertility. If a child talks to me about 'Enrico', this may be the patient's brother (historical reference), a split-off part of the patient, a name for the analyst, a split-off part of the analyst, etc. But if I leave the name 'Enrico' alone and consider it a *functional aggregate*, it becomes all this as well as a signal that the pair is functioning in a particular way, a mode which needs 'Enrico' on stage in order to be expressed. We could be dealing, for instance, with a warm, intimate atmosphere in the functioning of the analytic couple which is 'named' through the appearance of 'Enrico'.

Bezoari and I (1992) had this in mind when we coined the term 'functional aggregate' : the emergence, in the analytic dialogue, of images, characters and narrative sequences which, by appearing, changing and dissolving, create animated holograms, the different ways of relating in the session.

These holograms, like the images of a joint dream, confer upon the characters of the dialogue the value of an initial level of shared symbolization in which the emotional field and the elements that move about in it are represented. Through successive transformations these experiences generate affects and meanings which become more precisely definable.

From this point of view the analytic couple speaks *only and always* about itself and about its mutual functioning. All the other possible levels, which *obviously and necessarily* exist from other vertices (the phantasy level of the patient only, the mythical and real levels of the patient's history, etc.) are entirely valid, as a sort of third component with respect to the couple, even though this third-party function is already performed by the setting and by the 'characters' in the session. At this point we must not forget what has already been said about the need for a hierarchy in the codes and models

161

operating at the same time, to help us understand what is happening in the session.

I would add one final comment concerning the role that is to be assigned to the 'story' and the 'narrative'. While the microstories that are developed in the session keep to the patient's communication and to the analyst's reverie in the here and now of the session, they combine to form a single story which has to be shared and built up together.

The 'story' (meaning both referential history and the history of the couple) guarantees both separation and duality. On the one hand this story functions as a mythical depository on which the transference draws; on the other hand it is also the place where the transference, once transformed by the relationship, returns to store itself and to structure that mythic continuity which lies at the base of the sense of identity. Just as splitting and 'characters' answer the need to space out affects and psychic events, so the 'story', which effectively distributes affects along a time axis, permits the mental and emotional facts to be assigned dates.

The analyst, too, uses the story as a sort of 'left luggage office' where he can leave the day's psychic events to decant and settle, when they bear weighty, unresolved relational and countertransferential implications. This is what happens when we say to a patient, 'You had an X type of relationship with your mother', while omitting to search for where, perhaps in a place hidden from us, that type of functioning we are describing is to be found in the present. After all, even Verne's Michele Strogoff had to show that he was blind before he could regain his sight.

Todorov (1971), in his discussion of the detective novel, examines successively the *mystery*, the *crime novel* and the *suspense novel*. The first is characterized by the presence of two stories, that of the crime and that of the investigation. The characters of the second story do not act; they just gather information. Moreover, since they lie outside the first story, nothing can happen to them. Indeed, it is very unlikely that the investigator will be threatened or hurt, let alone killed. We have here two stories of which one is absent, but real, while the other is present, but not significant. In Todorov's classification, the crime novel follows a very different model: the two stories are fused, or rather, the first story is eradicated by the second. The crime being investigated does not take place prior to the narrative, since action and narrative coincide. Here there is no mystery, no enigma, and curiosity is replaced by suspense. The situation takes shape as the narrative proceeds; anything is possible and the investigator runs palpable risks, even his life may be in danger. So the second story, that which unfolds in the present, is put in the foreground. Todorov then goes on to describe a third category: the suspense novel. This one, like the mystery, has an enigma and a two-story structure, one past and the other present, but it does not reduce the second story to a mere gathering of facts. It is the second one, in fact, that is more significant. Curiosity about the past is retained, but what is much more important is the suspense about what is going to happen. The mystery is only a starting point, and it is the second story in which the real interest lies. Furthermore, the investigator loses his immunity and is exposed to all sorts of dangers. It is this last model which, applied to the question of the 'story' in psychoanalysis, seems to me the most creative. It is completely different from aseptic monopersonal analysis, with its reconstructions, its structures investigated and uncovered by a Poirot-like analyst; different too from the tendency towards fusion which denies separation and difference not only in the stories but also in the experiences and the affects of the minds.

I am speaking here of a 'story' which is true from an emotional point of view and is therefore subject to continual adjustments and transformations, as Barale points out (1990) with his reference to the microstories waiting to be thought, or rather, awaiting other possible meanings which are momentarily obstructed by the prevailing story, lying there like unsaturated potentialities of the internal world.

Of course in the session there is an oscillation between the 'story' and the 'relationship'. Just as we respect the patient's splitting, so we respect his dislocations in time, while remaining aware that the feelings exist only in the present, and that it is only these that can be known, as Bion so often reminds us. I believe, however, that the 'thermal shields' of splitting and of time must be respected as the guarantors of the affective universe of the patient (and of the analyst). If we ignore these, we will find ourselves either with two irreconcilable and incommunicable nuclei or with the indistinctness of undifferentiated material.

We find an example of a 'memory' occupying a different place in the 'story' in a clinical case cited by Miller (1981). Miller reports about patients who constantly, uncontrollably invade the private lives of their analysts by telephoning at night. Instead of pointing out to the patient that he feels too frustrated at having to wait for the next session, or that he has other failings (according to the structural model), the authoress suggests that we should be able to detect how patients' behaviour represents a re-enactment of an experience they suffered at the hands of their parents. To illustrate this point Miller notes how, after one of these interpretations, the distant recollection of a trauma found expression. The patient's father was a successful artist and regularly came home late, when his daughter was already asleep. He liked to get her up and play wonderfully exciting games with her until he got sleepy. Then he would put her back to bed, expecting her to fall asleep again. But, I ask myself, why not reverse this vertex and think of this scene as a detailed description of how the girl experiences the analytic hour and the functioning of the two minds in the session? In other words, the girl experiences an analyst arriving late and appearing too excited. The result is that he is perceived as in need of a discharge. Indeed, after awaking and 'exciting' the girl patient, he leaves her alone again and disappointed. Why not learn in the present about how to approach the patient, about how to interpret in such a way as to achieve a different effect? Perhaps the effect of so exciting an analyst might come precisely from his availability to receive the patient's projective identifications that make him that way; a way which, must be rethought and transformed in the analyst's working-through, before a new and different story can be told.

But we discussed this in Chapter 5 on dialogue, models of the mind and the status of characters in the analytic session.

The analyst's mind at work: problems, risks, needs

As I stated in Chapter 1, and tried to show in subsequent chapters, the analyst's mind is deeply involved in the relationship with the patient and plays an active role in determining, or rather helping to determine, what goes on in the field. His mind is continually exposed to beta elements, to the patient's projective identifications, and to the analyst's own natural PS$\longleftrightarrow$D oscillation. This leads to a series of consequences.

Safeguarding the patient

A first requirement: we must not pollute the patient's mind, and we must be truly willing to give him 'a place' inside us (Di Chiara 1985).

There are, of course, physiological splits, or better 'cleavages', that allow us, within certain limits, to keep outside the consulting room those mental states that may interfere in our work with the patient. But it is far from true that these systems always work. It is not unlikely, then, that we ourselves may invert the flow of projective identifications towards the patient (Di Chiara 1983; Nissim Momigliano 1984; Ferro 1987a, b), or at least shield ourselves with an analgesic mental attitude. This makes us unavailable to receive the patient's projective identifications, which then boomerang back at him in amplified form.

We should not take for granted that we can always be in touch with 'our share of mental suffering'. (As I will explain in greater detail below, this suffering may be *ours* due to particular, unavoidable internal or external circumstances, but also because we are disturbed or invaded by a particularly serious or invasive patient, and occasionally our suffering may be provoked by the patient himself in the course of a session.) It is essential not only to be aware of this possibility but also to gather information from the field about how we are functioning. Ultimately, the field, and what happens in it, serves as an instrument panel of our mental functioning.

Every time we receive a signal (or have the sensation) that we are functioning poorly, we must search for the causes (and countertransference dreams are extremely valuable to this end). We must immediately begin working once again at metabolizing the anxieties we have introduced into the field. After all, if, as Bion says, the analysis is a twofold affair, the risk is unavoidable, if only for the fact that we too are alive.

Quite often it is the patient herself who helps the analyst regain contact with his own mental functioning, and only when this functioning becomes adequate again will it be possible to continue the journey together.

It should not be assumed that a disturbance in functioning is necessarily due to interpretive inadequacy. The opposite may be the case, especially in the event that the crossing of projective identifications shifts to the disadvantage of the patient.

A few examples

Distrust of the roadworkers

Marcella, a girl who had not produced much at the Wednesday session, brings in a dream on Friday. She had to meet up with her mother and with a friend. Instead she found herself in a bus with some elderly people who were going to an island. There were two roadworkers clearing up a landslide.

After a few comments of mine, Marcella introduces an *anxious boy*. The boy is very jealous of his sister and locks Mother and Father in the bathroom. Then he ties string all over the house.

Marcella is pointing out that in the preceding session the encounter she had hoped for did not take place. Instead, she found herself in a different situation.

Instead of picking up just on this 'emotion' I focus on details of the meaning of the dream, and it is this that creates (as the two minds spin and weave together) the boy who arranges ropes-bonds-details to close off access to meanings rather than establish a relationship of trust with the two road maintenance workers already present in the field.

When it is possible to 'become aware in time': the bars in the window

During a session with a psychotic boy with violent projective identifications, I found myself having the following phantasy: I shouldn't live in a ground floor flat any more, with all those windows that are so easy to get

166

in through. Either I'm going to a higher floor or I'm going to put bars on the windows. Otherwise burglars could break in, and how awful it would be if someone turned my flat upside-down. Maybe it would be an idea to get a gun.

This phantasy clearly represents a barrier and a shield against the patient's emotions, which are felt as too invasive. But it also expresses hatred for the patient (Winnicott 1949), who with his projective identifications makes a mess of my mind and makes me feel robbed. What is more, it reveals a plan to invert the flow of projective identifications toward the patient himself by shooting at him the anxiety he had activated inside me.

Muscle or head?

Marco, a 4-year-old boy, gives a good idea of what these concepts mean in a drawing of his mother. She is incapable of opening up to his emotional needs and immediately saturates his concrete requirements: an arm is drawn in the place of her head, a bulging muscle where the receptive mind should be. Later, in a game, the child seems to suggest that unless the projective identifications are received and contained, unless they encounter reverie or availability-permeability (the precondition for reverie), they return in enlarged form and become increasingly destructive (Bion 1962; 1967c). But the same thing happens if the patient does not find in the analyst a mind-space capable of receiving, holding in and transforming, before interpreting (Alvarez 1985).

Rosenfeld (1987) speaks of the need not only for the right interpretation but also for the right opening of the mind. Of course, we also receive signals when sessions go well and when effective communication is resumed.

Gianluca's open bucket

A quite different case, it seems to me, is that of Gianluca, a 14-year-old boy who has been in analysis for two years. When he feels received and understood, Gianluca depicts the face and head of his analyst as a bucket without a lid, an open, receptive container-head (Lussana 1992a). I believe this corresponds to Riolo's suggestion (1983), that the analyst should receive 'all' the projective identifications coming from the patient.

Hautmann (1965) on the other hand reminds us that for Bion projective identification represents an ongoing process in the therapeutic relationship and that the good mother is able to take in her child's anxieties.

167

The confluence of rivers: Marcella

Marcella again, after a very intense session, comes out with the following dreams: There was a confluence of two rivers. The two became one. Then she found some wonderful sweets.

A boy was keeping guard at a castle. Marcella was going home. A woman was giving birth. The woman's legs were like the confluence of the rivers.

She was going to her bedridden grandmother's house. She looked after her affectionately.

The dreams signal the spinning and weaving of a shared meaning and ongoing repair work.

Lucia's 'dandelion leaves'

This is how Lucia signalled a moment of tranquillity, intimacy and good functioning: There was an open-air lunch. The various dishes were garnished with tender, bright green 'dandelion' leaves. Her friend Dino arrived. He was a cook and waiter, had a degree in medicine, and was modest but well respected. Lunch was served on a table made of warm, intensely veined cherry wood. Massimo came with some exciting Brazilian music. Then it was time to go, leaving mother and father with broken hearts. Ther train was about to leave and couldn't be missed.

This dream signals many transformations that have taken place from the time when Lucia's excessive reserve made it difficult for her to progress towards the capacity to think.

Inversion of flow and the oscillating gradient of projective identifications

I will now deal in somewhat greater detail with the inversion of flow of projective identifications. I have already discussed the question from a relational point of view and will reproduce parts of that paper (1987a). I will then follow with some observations from a field perspective which I consider more up to date.

Considering the relationship

Let's see if the literature can help us to formulate the concept with precision. Winnicott (1949) reports how at a particular point he realized that he was doing a poor job. He was making mistakes with all his patients and he recognized that this was due principally to the high level of tension he had attained with a particular psychotic patient. Money-Kyrle (1956) gives a careful description of the processes of introjection and projection that the analyst carries out with the patient and of the difficulties he encounters when the patient represents something that he has not yet learned to comprehend rapidly. Money-Kyrle shows that when the situation becomes intolerable, the analyst may make defensive projections and, together with the patient, may project aspects of himself. He then describes how the patient's projective identifications contribute to the creation of emotional disturbances in the analyst and the effects these disturbances may have on the patient.

In another publication Money-Kyrle (1978) reports a patient's dream in which a washing machine that used to work quite well suddenly reverses function and instead of cleaning clothes, soaks them in dirty water. The author recognizes that at that moment his own understanding was defective.

Brenman (1977), recognizing the advances made by Bion, considers obsolete the view according to which projective identifications were regarded as operating in only one direction.

Meotti (1984) points out that not only concepts and theories but also 'the analyst's moods' may be superimposed on the patient's material and argues that this may occur when the analyst is in poor shape, tired or uneasy. He adds that even a good mother, if she is mentally occupied, may make use of her own child to pour into him what she finds difficult to contain in herself.

Miller (1979) remarks that these children could become good analysts, though they may have the tendency to do with their patients what their mothers did with them. One such child was Marcella (discussed below), an adolescent who dreamt she was a vacuum cleaner and had to metabolize everything in the environment, including her analyst's mind.

We are speaking about the inversion of the flow of evacuative projective identifications. A good example of this is the 'green hand' discussed by Di Chiara (1983), who, like Ogden (1979), regards errors in technique as possible projective identifications of the analyst.

At this point some clarification is necessary. Since, as Manfredi Turillazzi (1985) notes, the concept of projective identification has become a sort of 'umbrella' covering a variety of phenomena, I want to make clear which sense of the term I am using. Projective identification is not something that occurs only in the phantasy; it may cause another person to have certain feelings.[1]

To help define the concept I will quote the words of a patient who seems to give a good description of what happens to me and inside him (since, as Meltzer says, projective identification may also take place inside one's own internal object). The boy says to me: 'You want to feel good. What about me? Until I've got somebody who cares about me and until I can care about someone, I can't let you go. You forget me with all my pain. So to hold on to you and to *force you and the others* to worry about little me *I have to send you some 'things'*: thoughts, fears, anxieties that *make you feel bad*. That way you're *obliged* to worry about me.' But let's go back to what I was saying before.

Langs (1984) asserts that much of the clinical material brought by patients does not originate solely in the intrapsychic conflict but may be considered an unconscious response to erroneous therapeutic interventions.

Nissim Momigliano (1984), too, discussing the circularity of the analytic dialogue, refers to projective identifications towards the patient and to their importance in the communication of the analytic pair.

I believe that this phenomenon, although undesirable, occurs more often than we think. They are the 'bad sessions', the patients that say they 'ate spoilt meat and vomited', the situations in which we are not sufficiently in contact with our own countertransference. Luciano, for example, is a patient with a serious disorder. He describes a (female) friend as a hollow piston (suggesting that I do not receive his projective identifications, or that I am even defending myself?). Then I have a dream in which there are strange, bizarre animals resembling rat-spiders. Feeling threatened, I cruelly massacre them all (the rejection of beta-elements?). Luciano (aware of this rejection?) begins to intrude violently into my life, telephoning me and apparently asking for help, but actually expressing protest and hatred. In the session I attempt to speak to the patient in a warm, gentle tone but instead send him my rage and aggressiveness. (I dream of troops that drive back terrorists and then invade their territories.) This goes on until I come into contact with my hatred, which I finally allow to surface in a stern tone of voice and in a new quality of interpretations. In this way I become more receptive and willing to accept the patient's beta-elements, and Luciano stops telephoning.

I am not concerned here with a single situation. I would prefer to divide the question into three parts. In the first and second I will describe two extreme situations which seem to me to establish the parameters for reflection, situations that are both connected with my own precarious mental functioning. In the third part I hope to show that what is seen in amplified form in the first two can occur, and I believe does happen, in more normal sessions as well.

The first case is related to a difficult personal situation in which I found myself. The second is connected with the massive projective identifications arriving from a very seriously disordered patient who, once again with vacation approaching, activated a psychotic transference. The patient's violent evacuations remained fixed in my mind and threatened to destroy it, until I managed to 'dissolve', through self-analysis or dreams, these 'pieces' that were stuck inside me.

But what happens to our patients (and, I would add, to our patients as a group) when our minds function poorly? Allowing the clinical material to speak for itself, I would like to stress that each patient reacts in his or her own way. Some, in fact, are able to carry out the operation described by Rosenfeld whereby they dream the split-off parts of the analyst's mind and help him to re-establish contact with those parts.

Which functions are the first to get hampered? The most 'sensitive', the ultimate and most complete expression of the analyst's proper mental functioning, is probably the reverie. Consequently, that is the first to go. Next, I believe, is the capacity for containment (Ferro 1985c). Subsequently, we find the analyst feeling persecuted and needing to evacuate beta-elements: those arriving from the patient but also the analyst's own.

Inversion when the analyst has personal problems

The following reports come from a period in which my mental presence was reduced, due to certain personal difficulties explained below.

I went to check what was written in the notebooks I keep for each patient and was dissatisfied with what I read. (Here I limit myself to what happened with the children in analysis.)

Gianluca

The boy was psychotic and had been in analysis for a year. This report dates from the middle of the period under examination. Coinciding with the period in which I am 'less present', Gianluca starts holding back his urine and excrement again. (Is his mother unable to metabolize the boy's beta-elements?) Once again he is terrorized by dirt. He keeps back 'torments and ugly things' because he is afraid that I cannot concern myself with them. And anyway, he is afraid that they are ugly and dirty. These 'things' are the hatred and rage he feels for his father 'who keeps him at a distance from his mother' on the days when I 'hinder' his coming to the session.

The analyst with a reduced capacity for reverie is perceived as a father who keeps him from discharging and from finding a receptive mother. Since I am less present, I do not allow him to have good sessions.

A few dreams will help to clarify the situation. 'I had two dreams,' says Gianluca. 'In the first there was me and another person. The other person was throwing poop at me, and dirtying me with pee. I had to respond.' At the time I interpreted this as his feeling my words were aggressive. Now I believe that he was speaking to me about the inversion of projective identifications, directed from me to him, since he felt that the period in

171

which he found my mind receptive was a thing of the past, as shown in Figure 8.1. At the top of the sheet Gianluca had written the following words: 'This landscape has caught fire (referring to the little town at the bottom) and everyone is running away, looking for other houses. After a bit the firemen come and put the fire out with water. The people who lived there before lost everything *and they went into other people's houses to find refuge, because they had no other choice.'*

Then there is the second dream: 'I was driving along a road and I got lost. I was alone, and then there were some other people who attacked me, with poop again.'

The container does not do its job. The patient is alone, and then bombarded. The analyst, who thought he could work and stand his own anxiety, was 'felt' by the patient as having precarious mental functioning, and the patient was a boy who had continually served as a rubbish bin for his mother's anxieties.

When I regain my tranquillity and start working again with good mental structure, the patient says: 'I was still thinking of coming with an umbrella, but I don't think it's necessary any more.' He no longer needs to protect himself from the beta-elements arriving from the analyst.

During one session a fuse blows and the lights go out. I interrupt the session to change it. When I return Gianluca says: 'I thought the fuse box exploded because of the rain. I was happy you fixed it, but angry because you left the room. But now let's go back to the dream I was telling you about.'

This is a comment on what happened. The analyst had an emotional jam, he exploded, he left, and then the analytic couple could get back to work. Perhaps this sequence could be seen as the overlapping of an internal situation of the patient and an internal situation of the analyst. It could also serve to raise the question of having to distinguish whether there was a genuine inversion or the realization of a negative transference connected with the patient's poor representations.

But in a situation as delicate as this, I feel that only the counter-transference can delimit the two cases, and in mine I had the distinct sensation that I was directly responsible for Gianluca's negative transference.

Marcella

The patient immediately picks up on my lack of presence in a dream: 'It was as if everything was still. There was an arcade. There was a lot of movement, with people going to and fro. There were stalls where they sold flowers, but there was no one there. I waited and asked around.'

Marcella seems to be well aware of the inversion of the child–mother functioning. It also appears that in her story she has made her mind available to her depressed mother.

Figure 8.1

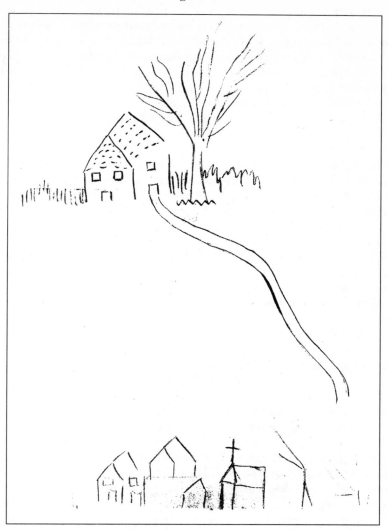

In connection with the next dream I can scarcely avoid recalling Rosenfeld, who says that certain patients have the capacity to dream the split-off parts of the analyst's mind at a particular moment. This seems to me proof that an inversion of projective identifications has taken place. 'In front of a school I see two dead children; it's as if they're in pieces, but there isn't any blood. They're in pieces, as if they were broken. Maybe they've been dead for many hours, or maybe they're dolls.' The patient told me this dream with detachment, as though it came from far away and did not belong to her.

After pondering over a number of different interpretive hypotheses, none of which I found satisfactory, I realized that Marcella had dreamt the deepest and most concealed anxiety I was suffering at that moment: dead children, though without blood; mentally dead, dolls, just as I felt my new-born daughters were. My children were being treated mechanically, serially, in the paediatric ward. Of course, I could think of the sterility of the couple, of our lifelessness as a couple at that moment, but how could I avoid considering the 'content' as well?

Needless to say, this dream helped me to decide, despite the doctors' opinion, to take my daughters out of that ward. The patient seems to have had a sort of reverie which delivered my anxious experience back to me.

Today I would say that, given the level of personal suffering, I should have suspended work, and that perhaps by continuing I was clutching at work in a period of difficulty.

Does this mean that every time the analyst has personal or family problems he should suspend work? Perhaps. Or should he or she be able to govern splitting, despite what happens within, in such a way that his distressed state does not interfere with the analysis? I do not believe that this is possible, because the question arises: where do the split-off parts go in such cases? Some end up in the patients' minds, I'm afraid.

Inversion caused by the relationship with a disturbing patient: the bites of the 'dragline bucket'

The second situation seems to me more problematic: the analyst is invaded by beta-elements, as frequently occurs with patients with serious mental disorders.

This is the case of Luciano, mentioned above. Luciano alternates periods in which work proceeds well with periods that are absolutely terrible, both for him and for me. When I am unable to transform and return to him his deepest anxieties, such dreadful moments occur without my realizing immediately that I have been invaded. This puts me in a difficult situation, which at times captures me and creates anxiety. I would like to describe one of these moments. In the Tuesday session, Luciano's terribly destructive part is at work (the 'grab' from a dream that attacked not only our relationship but also both our minds). I was prey to the fear, the panic, the terror of being attacked, and it was of little use to work on these things, since the teeth of the clamshell bucket (= 'benna' = 'belva'? [wild beast]) were real and attacked my mind.

I had regarded this part of the patient for some time as a *parasite* with metal jaws, who could never be satiated since it took its fill and emptied out everything. But while this biting was going on, what happened with the other patients?

It might be appropriate to recall that Costa (1979), considering patients as a whole, regards them as an internal object. De Simone Gaburri *et al.* (1981), speaking of groups, also stress that internal objects may move within the internal–external space of the group and from the group to the individual and vice versa.

Francesco

The boy is 8 years old and has been in analysis for two of them. He seems to take responsibility for the situation. After making an origami figure (an owl) he almost has a reverie: those were the days, when they would sit in the kitchen, he cutting and folding figures and his mother next to him sewing. He seems to be saying that times were good when he felt the analyst present, working together with him.

At the height of the 'clamshell bucket' invasion I forget to put the customary cushion on Francesco's chair. The following day, at the beginning of the session, Francesco makes a lot of origami figures, but they either 'fly or live in the water'. I point this out to him. 'Yes, it's as though there had been an earthquake and the animals had fled the land to seek refuge in the air or in the water.'

If the analyst is less present, if he falls prey to an emotional earthquake, the only way out is to seek refuge in madness and depressive inertia. Francesco begins the next session speaking about the 'fizzy' sensation he felt in his eyes (the desire to cry). When I suggest that he is afraid of feeling neglected and disappointed, he constructs a Saint Bernard with a flask attached to its collar, bringing warmth to the aid of someone trapped beneath an avalanche and freezing to death.

I would like to raise a few questions at this point. What should the analyst do in a situation like this? I do not believe that cancelling the sessions would be a solution in this case. Should he have such a capacity to metabolize beta-elements that he does not interfere in the patient's mental life? Unfortunately, this is not always possible.

Perhaps he should continue to take care (painfully) of the patient-children as suggested by Francesco's nostalgic vision of the son who is cutting paper alongside the mother who is sewing. In other words, he should continue repairing despite the attacks and persecution (Meotti and Meotti 1983).

On occasion, when the patient has showed that he is aware, I have confirmed that I am in fact 'less present mentally', though without going into detail or making countertransferential confessions. Then I proceed to interpret.

But what effect do my words of confirmation have? In general relief and worry. I must say, though, that even on those occasions when I did not feel I could give explicit confirmation, the patient still managed to overcome *my* difficult moments.

Which of the two approaches results in less suffering and more trust in the relationship depends, I believe, on the specific situation and on the stage of the analysis. Moreover, each patient seems to react in his or her own way to the analyst's reduced presence, a way that is determined by the patient's own early relationships.

Another problem is that of the passage, via the analyst's mind, of projective identifications from one patient to another, with their subsequent return to the analyst. As a marginal note we might also ask ourselves to what extent the inversion of flow which is not controlled and not understood but acted out, also by means of acting out interpretations, might lead to negative therapeutic reactions or psychotic transference (De Masi 1984; Barale and Ferro 1992; Gagliardi Guidi 1992).

Inversion in the normal course of work

This seems to me at once the most important and the most difficult situation to clarify. Perhaps the problem could be formulated like this: is the analyst's alpha function a constant or does it too have vicissitudes which may under certain circumstances go as far as inversion and under other circumstances go only as far as to hamper the function itself?

Bion speaks of this inversion in patients on more than one occasion, and Meltzer (1978b) has devoted a paper to the question of the disturbance of alpha function. Is it the upsetting of the analyst's alpha function that causes the inversion of the flow of projective identifications?

For Meltzer the inversion of direction (functioning) of the alpha function is compatible with the treatment of thoughts by evacuating them. If the capacity to think thoughts is missing (or is attacked), there may still be the capacity to try to rid the mind of thoughts (in the same way as it frees itself of excess stimuli). There would be a disassembly, according to Meltzer. The dream-thoughts, the unconscious thoughts during the waking state that represent the fabric of the contact barrier, would be transformed into alpha-elements, stripped of all the characteristics that distinguish them from beta-elements, and, finally, they would be projected.

There might be some less than macroscopic upsetting of the (analyst's) alpha function that is sensed by the patient, and by certain patients in particular (those patients, that is, whose parents' alpha function had been similarly upset: those children who 'took care of' their parents). There might be those 'wrong interpretations' (or interpretations insufficiently thought through) and moments of non-comprehension (derived from this minor compromise of the analyst's alpha function which could occur in more 'normal' sessions), that the patient feels as punctures, penetrations, needles, that is, as small quantities of beta-elements striking him. Let's take a closer look.

Maurizio

Maurizio is in his third year of analysis. He is 13 years old. At the Tuesday session, the second of the week, Maurizio tells me about his worries concerning his 'motorcycle', towards which he feels the love one has for a primary object. When he expresses his concern about being separated from it, because someone 'might get close with a screwdriver and ruin it for him', I give a credible interpretation.

In the course of the session I give other credible, but 'theoretical' interpretations, that is, not interpretations that arise there and then in the relationship but ones that come to my mind ready-made. I draw back from the anxieties about damage the patient has regarding his work with me. I do not receive his communication and metabolize it. Rather, I use mannered interpretations to evacuate into him anxieties about damage that he has activated in me. I also deny persecutory guilt in connection with this damage.

Consequently, there is not merely an absence of reverie, but there is also an inversion of the flow of projective identifications. No, I cannot make room for this anxiety. I deny access to it. But this anxiety evokes in me anxieties with which I am not, at the moment, in contact. By speaking to you about other things, it is I who evacuate my anxieties into you.

The therapist, then, uses the patient to free himself of something of his own. In other words, he does not merely respond to the patient's feeling, perhaps by acting it out, but he discharges something of his own into the patient.

There is no session on Wednesday, and Maurizio does not come to the session on Thursday. At this point, I begin to think about what happened during the Tuesday session, and I realize with dissatisfaction that the interpretation I gave was lifeless. On Friday Maurizio arrives late. As I wait for him to arrive, I find myself having phantasies about a possible accident he might have had, connecting it with the Tuesday session.

When he finally arrives, it is unclear whether he is more manic or angry. He tells me about an accident he had with a car which forced him to jump: the motorcycle was destroyed but he was left unhurt. I feel my flesh creep.

Smiling, he tells me it was a joke. It didn't really happen. But something had tormented him enormously. The fear that someone, maybe his father or mother, might have poured something into the fuel tank of his bike, not the right proportion of oil to obtain the correct mixture but detergent, cognac or alcohol.

At this point it is not difficult for me to interpret his worry that in the Tuesday session, rather than helping him with interpretations that facilitated good functioning, he felt I was damaging him with what I said. My interpretations were inappropriate, like detergent or alcohol, and ruined his mind-engine.

Maurizio answers quickly and without hesitation that this is true, and that it may have been due to these worries that he skipped the session on Thursday. This gives us the opportunity to examine the fear of a crazy analyst-mother who, instead of metabolizing her child's mind, damages it. Maurizio adds: 'A mother that doesn't give you fresh things but . . . I don't know . . . rotten eggs from the fridge.'

During the session we also have occasion to note what the patient was wearing that day: a jacket like a bulletproof vest. And we work on the patient's phantasy about the consulting room being full of the analyst's guns, all aimed at him. As a consequence the patient feels the need to keep the fuel tank of his mind-bike locked because he is afraid that he cannot be too trusting.

What the patient has reactivated (or perhaps I should say what the patient and analyst have reactivated thanks to criss-crossing projective identifications) is also his early experience with a seriously psychotic mother. I believe that Maurizio was recounting and reliving the bombardment of beta-elements from his mother, a mother whose mind could certainly not be open to metabolizing through reverie, but who on the contrary used her son as the impossible container of her own intolerable anxieties.

The internal situation of the analyst cannot be considered invariant but must be continually rearranged. This holds, provided that the analyst does not take refuge in a fortress of theories, using them as a justified defence against contact with his patient, and that his analytic equipment is adequate (Greenson 1967; Di Chiara 1982).

The analyst, then, must continually work on his own mental structure, reconstituting it by paying constant attention to the countertransference. He must work on recovering a psychoanalytic function of the mind (Hartmann 1985b), and a parental distance from the patient (De Martis 1983). This function and distance will be put to the test continually by the patient and by the collusions that may always be activated in the analyst (Di Chiara *et al.* 1985). It should be stressed that violent projective identifications, arriving from patients with serious disorders, may cause the analyst to act out under the internal pressures of which he himself may for some time be unaware. In the case of Maurizio, the analyst may truly function like a crazy or collusive mother until he realizes the anomalous and perverse aspects of the relationship (Ogden 1979). As I said earlier, the patient's response to the therapist's projective identifications will vary according to the early relationships he had.

There are patients who even have the capacity to metabolize these projective identifications (those who cared for their parents' minds) or who at any rate do not seem to be particularly disturbed by them. Once, after a session in which I had made many mistakes in timing and pacing, the patient simply told me that she had been to a fashion show with her mother and that she could not understand why all the handbags and shoes were out of place. 'But you know how it is with these shoemakers.'

To summarize, I have tried to describe the inversion of the flow of projective identification in three situations: an analyst overloaded with as yet unmetabolized anxieties; an analyst violently intruded on by a particularly disturbing patient; and an analyst working normally in whom, however, parts kept distant can always be ready to interfere in the relationship with the patient.

I should make it clear that I am not speaking of the projective identifications which the analyst uses to communicate. The analyst, after all, like any other human being, may resort to projective identification as a normal way of communicating (Bion 1962; Di Chiara *et al.* 1985). Rather, I am speaking of those characterized by their 'sting' or by the 'discharging' qualities, in other words, those that are evacuative. This kind of projective identification must be considered as relative, for much depends on the capacity of the container to remain unharmed.[2]

In this connection we might recall what Leonardi wrote (1987): 'The patient with whom we are not in contact, that is, the one we receive in our mind inadequately . . . is a falsification deriving from our projective identifications, evacuating what he is at that specific moment, perhaps reducing him to what he was a year or a week before . . . Our thought is a stereotype originating not in the truth of an emotional message, but in a programme that uses our mental apparatus as though it were a computer.' One might ask whether in such cases what is evacuated is only the actual patient or whether, with our computer–like interpretations, we are not also evacuating our unthought/unthinkable emotions.

Langs is right when he states that interpretations that are wrong in content are projective identifications towards the patient. Even more so are those that are defective in manner or timing, pacing and distance (Meltzer 1976), as well as those lacking tact, as Carloni (1984) would put it.

There is another element to consider: the quality of the receiver. It may depend on the receiver whether the analyst's mistaken interpretations provoke simply anger or catastrophic reactions.

179

Many interpretations may well be 'undigested' (thoughts that have not yet been sufficiently thought out), that is, impregnated with sensations and impressions as yet not entirely transformed into thoughts (Manfredi Turillazzi 1978). Perhaps it is the degree of beta–elements they contain that constitutes the evacuative projective identifications which make the neurotic patient feel overloaded and the psychotic invaded.

Mancia (1984) also proposes dividing dreams into those that work through and those that evacuate. He describes the latter as 'dominated by symbolic equations in which the symbolization is scarce or absent, and the 'alpha' function is inadequate to the alphabetization of the 'beta' elements, which are then evacuated.'

In the interpretation this seems to happen when the analyst is at work on his own split parts rather than on his parts in a situation of good distinction separation. A good interpretation, then, is the fruit of permeability, continence and reverie when one is in contact with one's own parts – even the most uncomfortable ones. Symbolic equations (Segal 1957, 1978), on the other hand, arise under the opposite conditions of impermeability, incontinence and the splitting of one's own parts.

At this point it could appear that we are running the risk of idealizing the analyst, and of possibly exaggerating his responsibility. But it should be remembered that if I have spoken at length about the analyst, this is because it is the analyst who is the subject of this section. But the analyst is just one of the poles of a couple, and it is the analytic couple that must always command our attention.

If what is evacuated is the suffering that thought cannot bear (Bion 1962), and if the result and purpose of splitting and projection is the exclusion of the unconscious vision of what produces pain (Meotti 1984), we can embrace the suggestion made by Vallino Macciò (1984) that we should rely less on verbal appearances and much more on the substance of our emotions, and that we should refine a method capable of unifying verbal thought with dream-thought.

Bion (1980) also reminds us that we must be aware that there are elements inside us about which we can do nothing. It is a matter of making the best of a bad deal. In this case we are the bad deal. No one can be analysed completely; there is no such thing. Eventually the analysis has to stop, and then we have to make do with what we are.

Considering the field

I have reproduced a considerable amount of my own work (Ferro 1987a) so as to illustrate a stage in my personal journey which led me to elaborate a concept of the field (meanwhile discovering that the notion was already outlined by the Barangers, Bion and Corrao). The point is that not only does the patient influence the analyst with all the problems connected with countertransference, but also the analyst, for the most varied reasons, influences the patient.

It is a short step from this recognition to considering the analytic situation as based on a common emotional field, the vectors of which are made up of cross–cutting projective identifications. The shifting of the gradient in one direction or another will determine the therapeutic efficacy of the situation for the patient. The following, however, are starting points:

1   In every analysis there will be 'disadvantageous' moments for the patient.
2   The emotional field is the result of combining the emotions of both members of the couple.
3   The analyst, with his own deep emotional state, conveyed by projective identifications, contributes to determining the field no matter how he behaves in the relationship: with his silences, his activity, his permeability, with all the oscillations of his mental functioning. The characters, as we have said, are from a certain vertex *the affective holograms of that functioning, a genuine three-dimensional fabric of the functioning of the couple.*

Safeguarding the analyst

This issue does not receive the attention it deserves. In reality the analyst is continually exposed to the patient's beta–elements, and the more permeable and mentally available he is, the more he takes on and transforms projective identifications, many of which are violent and toxic. The analyst then must consciously devote time to his own 'detoxification'.

An opposite approach is to shield oneself at times by continuous (pseudo-) therapeutic activity, which serves as a sort of 'leaden smock'. The patients find a place where their functioning is X-rayed, but never a place where they are thought about. This continuous activity is not unlike what Bick (1968) refers to as wearing a second skin.

Leaving aside the case of therapists who treat effort by mithridatizing themselves with further effort, we need to find a way to make good, continuous mental functioning possible. This, after all, is what Winnicott was referring to when he said that at the beginning of an analysis his aim was to remain awake and alive. Meltzer, too, stressed the need to safeguard the analyst through the setting.

What instruments can we use to achieve all this? First of all, there should be periods of rest: in the course of the year, vacations; during the week, weekends; during the day, free time, or moments devoted to other activities;

and finally that fountain of 'refreshment' which are the ten minutes necessary between one patient and another.

The diversification of activities also means programming not only the hours of therapy but also the time reserved for study, writing, seminars, conferences and meeting colleagues. Above all, we must know how to *stop being an analyst outside working hours and outside the setting* in order to get hold of other vertices again which are broader and can be shared.

Before taking up this point, I would like to repeat that counter-transference dreams are precious indicators of both our internal state and our mental labour. Though they are not limited to the 'instrument panel' function, they are also charged with metabolizing mental effort.

Connected with these observations is the problem of the criteria of analysability. The first requirement is to ascertain whether we have sufficient mental availability, health and strength to accept a given new patient.

Touching upon this question, I must of course broaden the view to include all the work the analyst does, that is, not only with children but also the work involving the entire group of patients.

A key question concerns to what extent we are willing to run risks in our everyday work, what the limit of risk is that we wish to approach, and how much we legitimately need to travel down safe, well-worn paths. This last area encompasses many questions pertaining to the criteria of analysability and the use of theories and models which have become defensive, though once they were revolutionary (Di Chiara 1991).

In any case, the analyst's mind, on condition that it is permeable, remains deeply implicated, and at times 'disturbed', in the relationship with patients (as long as the analyst does not seek refuge, like a radiologist, behind his 'leaden smock', thus blocking the penetration of the patient's emotions, and limit himself to interpreting the patient's functioning as though it were an invariable).

A few examples will illustrate the analyst's mental suffering. I have a dream. After having a CAT scan, I am told that I have two blood cysts in the brain: one rather high up and the other further down. Then there is a third one. These pockets of blood are rather dangerous and will require surgery. It may be necessary to do a carotid test, in itself rather dangerous, but it is also possible that simpler treatment will be enough. *In any case, it is something that requires serious attention.*

As soon as I wake up I feel struck by and curious about this dream. These contained, encapsulated micro-haemorrhages do not seem to compromise my mental functioning but I have to be concerned about them. I try to connect the dream with the events of my present or past life. It is a calm, productive period of my life. Despite my efforts, I cannot find any possible association. I am reminded of the end of an analysis and, at this point, remember another flash of the dream. The CAT scan also revealed scars of completely healed wounds. What does this mean?

Then a thought comes to mind that feels right. I am about to finish analysis with three patients: one in a few days and the other two in a few months, with dates already fixed. So for my mind the end of analysis of a patient, and the separation from him, implies micro-haemorrhages that, although circumscribed and contained, require my attention.

In this connection we could recall Klauber's (1979) complaint that there has been no discussion of how the analyst manages to establish quite intimate relationships with one patient after another, nor has attention been paid to the pain the therapist feels for each patient and how he discharges it.

It may be only in extreme situations (the analyst's acting out and projective identifications directed at the patient) that this pain is 'discharged'. Usually, I think, it is metabolized through self-analysis, contact with colleagues, scientific work (see Widloecher, quoted by Klauber 1979), and in certain moments through countertransference dreams.

Countertransference dreams are of vital importance. Not only do they help clarify the deep interrelationships of the analytic couple, but they also have the capacity to integrate and repair the analyst's mind and to metabolize his mental health.

Meltzer (1978a) points out that there are ways of remaining unaware of the pain inside the analyst. There are also systems for getting free of it by placing it in various objects of the external world. He cites Freud's clinical notes on the Rat Man as a case in point. Freud, he notes, realized that his patient was causing him pain, humiliating him, and provoking his anger by denigrating his love objects: his wife, his daughter and so on.

Let's see how the transference represents the behaviour of the 'cruel captain' the Rat Man speaks about. Meltzer (1978), once again, admires Freud's extraordinary patience and good humour. He notes how calmly Freud dealt with these manifestations of transference. On the basis of his theory, he saw them as revisions of past events and relationships which actually had nothing to do with him. But we can suppose, adds Meltzer, that Freud kept a certain distance from the material in order to protect himself from countertransferential involvement. Meltzer also notes, however, that Freud acted out part of the revulsion he felt for his patient (for example, by exchanging the patient's material with that of another patient).

Different functions of the analyst can suffer damage. A search for the most important could lead us to the insult that the Rat Man hurls at Freud (by way of the recollection of a childhood experience involving the patient's father): 'Lamp, plate, towel' (Freud 1909). Our approach will be to consider these insults as pertaining to the then and there of the relationship.

Freud tells us these are the words of a child, who, not knowing insults adequate to the task of expressing his rage, randomly chooses the names of objects. It is interesting, however (and amusing!) to consider them also as explicit references to the three principal functions of analysis. Each of these functions, depending on which theoretical model is employed, has been described in different ways and each, it seems, was already present in Freud. The 'lamp' can be seen as an allusion to light, to cognitive operations, to clarifying and finding meanings, ways of constructing and interpreting. The 'plate' recalls the nutritional function, and the 'towel' the absorbing, cleansing function – ranging from the toilet-breast (Meltzer) to reverie (Bion).

But the lamp can overheat and melt, the plate can crack or break, and the towel can become dirty, wet and unable to carry out its proper function. Of course, this reading is merely a humorous metaphor. But why not, if it helps clarify concepts and functions?

In the *Notes* to *Rat Man* we see how Freud (1909) employs scientific detachment and distance to protect the 'lamp', the 'plate' and the 'towel' from violent attacks. He describes a dream in which the patient is lying on his back on top of a girl (Freud's daughter), using the faeces dangling from his anus to copulate with her. The description of the dream is presented as 'a splendid anal phantasy'.

Would we be going too far if we suggested that the dream described what the patient was doing to the analyst at that moment, that is, launching a faecal attack, or a violent evacuative projective identification, via the daughter, towards the more receptive (♀) part of Freud himself?

Freud makes no mention of it, and he masks it behind that 'splendid anal phantasy', but where did the patient's violent evacuative projective identification end up? Somewhere other than in Freud's mind? If this is the case, that mind must have run the risk of overheating, breaking or at least getting dirty.

But we still have the problem of how the analyst tolerates all this and restores his own mind. In the midst of these considerations we find another phenomenon which has by now been recognized and described (Waksman 1985): the case of expert analysts who abandon the practice of child analysis and seek refuge in the supervision of analysis or child therapy (Siniavsky 1979). Various reasons have been suggested for this abandonment, including the mental, and sometimes physical, burden of work with children, the countertransferential difficulties in which the most archaic identifications are reactivated, and the greater need children have for real containment, which cannot be replaced by the analyst's authority.

But let's return to the period in which I had the 'blood cyst' dream. A few days later a patient, Luigi, has a dream in which he goes to a hospital to visit his father and mother for the last time, as they are both in the 'terminal phase'. He hugs them, cries and says how much he loves them. Present during all this there are some inattentive, uninterested doctors. The patient, by now in an advanced stage of analysis, poses these questions: certainly, he has feelings and is suffering because of the approaching vacation and the end of analysis; he is in mourning, as is clear from a series of dreams; but while he is crying and experiencing these deep feelings for his father and mother, what am I, the doctor, feeling for him? Am I merely presiding over the therapeutic rite, like a priest who, as soon as the funeral mass is over, lets his thoughts wander? Or am I participating directly in this experience with him? He doesn't think so, but my participation is the only thing that gives him the strength to experience emotions fully in the analysis.

In another publication (Bezoari and Ferro 1991b) I quoted a patient who said: 'Doctors want to stay healthy. They don't smoke, so it's up to me to do all the smoking.' Here the patient was saying that he felt alone in having to face intense, painful emotions and states of mind.

A dream helps indicate how risky it is to take on a patient with a serious disorder. I am holding a baby girl in my arms called 'Faith'. We have to be together. Then I am in a research laboratory, and I want to be inoculated with a dangerous virus. An assistant first strokes his beard and then stings my forearm (injects the virus). Then there is the head of the laboratory. He shows me a precious collection of vaccinations and cures, all requiring testing. It will take years. A young assistant, perhaps the daughter of the head of the laboratory, is worried and says: 'But why did you do it? As a doctor, for the sake of science?' 'No,' I answer, 'as a journalist.' 'That's not enough.' 'The truth is that I have a double identity: doctor and journalist.'

This dream reveals the activation of an internal work group: the need for 'Faith', or rather trust, a test of strength, the awareness of risk, and the fact that we analysts are at a crossroads between therapy and knowledge, between treating and narrating. Certainly, working without the safety net of super-organized theories means that repairs will be necessary, as Barale and I pointed out in the work on countertransference dreams.

Let us conclude this section with another illustration of the work which takes place beneath this interpretive activity, and which prepares for it. I will present two of my dreams that may be considered as 'work' on the patients but which could also describe the 'work' after taking on the patient's projective identifications.

1   There were some parasites and cocci that were growing into spiders. There were many of them, as in the film *The Invasion of Ultrabodies*. I was uncertain whether to stop them, kill them, or watch and let them grow.
2   The same night: a long stretch of a trip in Spain. It was very hot, with little refreshment. Suddenly there was a rainstorm. The car, which had been running well, broke down. The windscreen wiper stopped on my side (the driver's), while the other (on the passenger's side) remained working. I continue to drive in the dark, as if it were foggy. I manage to keep on the road. The weather improves quickly and the fog disappears.

I am looking for a mechanic, or at least a petrol station. There are far more than I had expected and I stop at one. It was the same one as many years ago. I ask a friend to see to the windscreen wiper. I open the boot and take out the tools. As I find a pair of pliers, some other people pull up. One of the passengers in the other car says he can help. He takes the circuitry apart, detaches and fixes the wires. I am very worried at the thought of the enormous amount of work we will have to do if he messes thing up. Fortunately, he manages to put the wires back in their place, and the circuitry functions well, at least as well as before. All I have to do is put things back together, and off we go again!

At this point the criteria of analysability are a function of the degree of risk and frustration to which the analyst is willing to expose himself. This is Meltzer's point when he says that we should not choose our patients and when he expresses the gratitude he felt toward the patients with serious disorders, even schizophrenics, who did several years of analysis with him. As an example, consider the analysis of a terminal patient or a microcephalous child as described by Vallino Macciò (1984, 1992).

I recall another dream which helped me set a limit on the number of working hours and determine the optimum composition of the group of patients, in terms of children, adults and patients with serious and less serious disorders. The suggestion proved necessary in order to avoid damaging others by *evacuating* elsewhere an excess of mental suffering.

A few pages back I mentioned the need to stop being an analyst outside working hours and outside the setting. This recommendation is particularly relevant to what will be said in the following section.

Safeguarding the family

This section picks up on a question raised in the preceding one concerning the destination of the anxieties and mental suffering of which the analyst himself may sometimes be unaware.

Marina, the 12-year-old daughter of a child therapist whom I consult, begins by saying: '*The real problem is that my mother is an analyst.*' She goes on to tell me about a catherine wheel of quarrels that often ignites: it is the catherine wheel of 'anger' that frequently involves the entire family and goes out only when the excess of tension has been released.

I was struck by her opening words, because I believe it is true that the analyst's work produces an accumulation of 'firedamp'. If this is not taken into account and if an ecological way of carrying it off is not found, it pollutes our mind and, in consequence, the minds of those around us.

But the people around us (just as I said about our patients) are also exposed to our *transformations in hallucinosis*, every time we try to exercise control over the real world and over the many vertices of that world by means of pseudo-interpretive activity. I say 'pseudo' because this activity is carried out beyond the setting. I remember one time I felt quite uneasy and opted for a much needed rest, when a close friend of mine told me his blood was low on iron, and I, thinking of my surname, immediately felt he was reproaching me for not coming to see him more often.

There are times when I have 'interpreted' the illness of my children or family members or what is said at social gatherings. These are all signs of the risk an analyst can run: a compulsory need to find connections and unambiguous, therefore false, explanations of the variety of human events. Only when the setting is established does the analyst have a right to carry out interpretive mental operations. Out of context we must, for the sake of our own mental health and that of others, constantly give up our interpretive instruments. In the same way, the surgeon is authorized to use a scalpel only when he works in the operating theatre. The same scalpel outside its setting not only 'infects' and 'contaminates' but becomes an instrument of offence or even death. Of course it is difficult for the analyst to free himself of the omnipotence he sometimes feels (just think of the reference of the patient's every communication in the transference). It is also difficult to face others with no particular equipment, as Freud reminds us when he says that, ultimately, analysis can only transform hysterical misery into common unhappiness.

Outside the setting, we are people who are simply more aware of how precious good mental functioning is. Outside the setting we will be that much 'richer' if we are able to be indistinguishable from everyone else. The finest compliment I have ever heard about a colleague was that, when off the job, at which he was very competent, 'no one would ever have guessed he was an analyst'.

'Wisdom comes to the learned man through the opportunities of free time.' Bion (1980) cites this verse from Ecclesiastes as he weighs the risks of knowledge against the benefits of wisdom.

Free time is 'for thinking'. This is the note on which I would like to end. We need free time in the session to relieve us of the pressure to interpret. We need free time between one patient and another, and between one period of work and another. Above all, we need free time to be with ourselves to find inspiration, freedom and awareness. It is this awareness that Bion evokes when he imagines being sent to heaven and finding a multitude of sheep, calves and birds that can prove they were all eaten by him. He is brusquely turned away and sent to hell, to be eaten. Eternal happiness is too much to expect, he concludes. As the song says, 'Love makes the world go round.' A realist searches for sources of energy (Bion 1980). I believe there is no better therapy than these thoughts against the idealization of ourselves and our work, and in favour of the passion and love necessary to continue our work in an inspired way. Among our patients, it is the children who most often force us both to listen to truths we would rather not hear and also to share passions and discoveries.

Notes

1 A review of the theoretical models

1 Of course, I am not calling into question the necessary differences in the setting and modes of expression. I am referring to the fact that the analyst's mental functioning is the same in various situations. For more on this see Flegenheimer (1983) and Wallerstein (1988). I am also speaking of realization and not application, for I am convinced that the so-called psychoanalytic lens is a *contact* lens, that is, it becomes effective only through the emotional contact between patient and analyst within a controlled setting.
2 Chapter 5 will present a detailed examination of a session with Richard.
3 In his discussion of the psychoanalytic functions of the analyst's mind, Di Chiara (1982) highlights the 'qualities' of contact and detachment, dependence and development, and attention. These qualities are obtained through the analysis of the analyst, which equips him with an 'analysed structure of the character'. See also Hautmann (1977), Carloni (1982) and (Greenson (1967).
4 It should be stressed, however, that there is an inclination to trace different tendencies in Freud (Chianese 1988; Muratori and Cargnelutti 1988).
5 The same central position that repression holds in Freud's model is held in Klein's model by the concept of splitting. Splitting is necessary to perform the first mental operations of discrimination, but if it is excessive parts of the self are lost.
   Bion's model focuses on the interrelationship between container and contained (♀ ♂). This implies that priority is given to relating with the other person who is the locus that gives life to the apparatus for dealing with thoughts. This operation involves the successful introjection of the relationship with the other mind, thus paving the way for the very capacity to think. This is made possible by repeating the communicative experience of the interplay between projective identifications and reverie.
6 This model considers facts described not as events of the internal world but as a reconstruction of historical events. This explains the different conceptions of the transference. For Klein, we are dealing with the outward projection of current phantasies, whereas Freud stressed the repetition of what could not be remembered.
7 Bion proposes a radical change in perspective on projective identifications. For him, projective identifications constitute the basic activity of the human mind in order to communicate emotions. He believes that the patient does something to the analyst and that the analyst does something to the patient (Bion 1980).

8 The conceptual innovations introduced by Bion, by the Barangers and by notions such as 'affective hologram' (Ferro 1991) and 'functional aggregate' (Bezoari and Ferro 1991b) completely overturn this point of view. The patient, knowing with whom he is dealing and how we function, using defences and being permeable or not to his projective identifications, structures the field just as much as the patient's way of presenting himself does. We must always bear in mind, however, that it is 'fundamental for psychoanalytic work' to have an instrument that is tuned well enough to be used with 'success' (Di Chiara 1982): the analysed mind of the analyst.

9 The depressive position is understood as a structuring of anxieties and defences, in which interest in and love for the object prevail. In Klein's view, the dominant characteristic of the depressive position was the recognition that love and hate are directed towards the same person. Segal stresses the connection between symbolism and the depressive position. Klein herself and Britton stress its intrinsic relation to the Oedipus complex. All Kleinian analysts stress not only love and hate for the same object, plus symbolism and the Oedipus complex, but also recognition of the object's separateness (Bott Spillius 1997, personal communication).

10 These concepts appear in Klein's *The Psychoanalysis of Children* (1932) and more systematically in *Our Adult World and Other Essays* (1959).

11 Bion used to say that you cannot be a Bionian, because adhering to a school of thought compromises the originality of your work as an analyst. Only the freedom and uniqueness of the analyst can guarantee fertility (Bion 1983; Bion Talamo 1987).

12 In this connection, it is interesting to recall the stages of this development as described by Meltzer (1967) in *The Psychoanalytic Process*: from the *realization of the transference to geographic confusion*, from *geographic confusion to zonal confusion*, then to the *thresholds of the depressive position* and finally *weaning*.

13 Bion's innovations were so revolutionary that they caused a 'catastrophic change' in the entire field of psychoanalysis, leaving no distinction possible between the analysis of children and adults. Klein also strongly implies that there is one psychoanalysis for both adults and children.

2 Drawings

1 After I gave this same patient an interpretation in which her two split parts were brought together prematurely, she had what I might call *a dream-like audio picture*, when she actually heard these two parts 'talking inside her head'.

2 I refer here, for the sake of simplicity, to the 'character', but the same is true of an articulated narration, a memory or an anecdote.

3 Play

1 One patient is very worried by a dream she has in which feathers are growing on her back. She is relieved when she realizes that she is simply calling herself a 'silly goose'.

2 This is how one mother presented her child to me: He had always been so well-behaved that she hardly even noticed his presence until he was 3 years old. At this age the child became seriously hyperactive. He has a game he plays which is always the same. There is a woman whose windows look out on the courtyard where the boy lives. The woman always keeps her shutters closed. The boy goes up to the

windows and bangs repeatedly on the shutters. Usually nothing happens, but every once in a while the woman opens the shutters and yells at the child. The boy begins the game again almost immediately. The mother also showed me a drawing. There is a truck, a car and a bicycle. All the vehicles seem to be going very fast, because there is a cloud of smoke at the exhaust pipe of each, and yet none has a driver. It seems to me that the child is very clearly expressing that there is a lack of willingness to take notice of him and to show him that there is a thinking mind present.

3 There are many examples of play interpreted symbolically in Aberastury (1981) and the meaning of every symbol is explained. But the author also stresses that it is necessary to grasp the whole situation each time – a doll may represent a penis, a boy the child himself, etc. In interpreting play we have to consider its representation in space, the traumatic situation it implies, and why it is here and now, in our presence, that the mood which accompanies the game is the root of every possibility of transformation.

4 In Italy, work has been done by Generali Clements (1971), Generali Clements and Ferrara Mori (1980), Ferrara Mori *et al.* (1981), Vallino Macciò (1981), Piontelli (1986), Lussana (1992a), Borgogno (1981), Di Cagno *et al.* (1981), Brutti (1975), Brutti *et al.* (1981), Negri (1987, 1991), etc.

4 Dreams

1 The reference here is to a character in an old TV commercial in which the Inspector, although infallible, went bald because he did not use a certain hair cream.

2 Orpioni: opiolionidi or falangidi (sic). Type of arachnid with short abdomen and very long legs, somewhat like a spider.

3 From Franz Kafka's *Metamorphosis*, translated by Willa and Edwin Muir, published by Penguin Books Ltd:

> As Gregor Samsa awoke one morning from uneasy dreams, he found himself transformed in his bed into a gigantic insect. He was lying on his hard, as it were armour-plated, back . . . His numerous legs, which were pitifully thin compared to the rest of his bulk, waved helplessly before his eyes . . . His room, a regular human bedroom, only rather too small . . . shutting his eyes to keep from seeing his struggling legs . . . He would have needed arms and hands to hoist himself up; instead he had only the numerous little legs which never stopped waving in all directions and which he could not control in the least . . . it struck him how simple it would be if he could get help . . . But . . . (Gregor was) condemned to work for a firm where the smallest omission at once gave rise to the gravest suspicion . . . he was eager to find out what the others . . . would say at the sight of him. If they were horrified . . . and [he] hoped for great and remarkable results from both the doctor and the locksmith . . . he heard the chief clerk utter a loud 'Oh!' and now he could see the man . . . clapping one hand before his open mouth and slowly backing away as if driven by some invisible steady pressure. His mother . . . first clasped her hands and looked at his father, then . . . fell on the floor . . . His father knotted his fist with a fierce expression on his face as if he meant to knock Gregor back into his room, then . . . covered his eyes with his hands and wept . . . (Gregor's) legs were completely obedient, as he noted with joy . . . his mother . . . cried: 'Help, for God's sake, help!' . . . there stood a basin filled with fresh milk in which floated little sops of bread . . . He dipped his head almost over the eyes straight into the milk. But . . . he did not like the milk . . . His parents . . . would not have wanted him to starve, but perhaps they could not have borne to know . . . about his

191

feeding . . . since what he said was not understood by the others, it never struck any of them . . . that he could understand what he said . . . Gregor's sole desire was to do his utmost to help the family to forget as soon as possible the catastrophe which had . . . thrown them all into a state of complete despair . . . made him realise how repulsive the sight of him still was . . . and that it was bound to go on being repulsive . . . he was fast losing any interest he had ever taken in food . . . Gregor was now cut off from his mother, who was perhaps nearly dying because of him . . . he began now to crawl to and fro over everything, walls, furniture and ceiling, and finally . . . in his despair fell down on to the . . . big table . . . He saw his mother rushing towards his father . . . as she begged for her son's life. Gregor was a member of the family, despite his present unfortunate and repulsive shape, and ought not to be treated as an enemy . . . family duty required the supression of disgust and the exercise of patience . . . (Gregor) was . . . filled with rage at the way they were neglecting him . . . and . . . would make plans for getting into the larder to take the food that was . . . his due . . . The cleaning of his room . . . could not have been more hastily done . . . Gregor was now eating hardly anything. Only when he happened to pass the food laid out for him did he take a bit of something in his mouth . . . and usually spat it out again . . . Anything that was not needed for the moment was simply flung into Gregor's room . . . in spite of his condition, no shame deterred him from advancing.

'We've tried to look after it and put up with it as far as is humanly possible . . . If this were Gregor, he would have realized long ago that human beings can't live with such a creature and would have gone away of his own accord . . . As it is, this creature persecutes us.'

'Just look at this, it's dead! . . . Now thanks be to God . . . Just see how thin he was. It's such a long time since he's eaten anything.'

At the end of their journey their daughter sprang to her feet first and stretched her young body.

8 The analyst's mind at work: problems, risks, needs

1 See Di Chiara and Flegenheimer (1985) for a discussion of the various positions on this subject.
2 This kind of projective identification must be considered as relative, for much depends on the capacity of the container to remain unharmed.

Bibliography

Abadi, M. (1987) 'Che cosa è interpretare', in Società Italiana di Psicoanalisi di gruppo (ed.) *L'interpretazione psicoanalitica*, Rome: Bulzoni.

Aberastury, A. (1981) *Teoria y técnica del psicoanalisis de niños*, Buenos Aires: Paidos.

Allen, W. (1986) ' The Kugelmass episode', in C.E. Bain (ed.) *The Norton Introduction to Literature*, New York: W.W. Norton, pp. 502–511.

Alvarez, A. (1985) 'The problem of neutrality: some reflections on the psychoanalytic attitude in the treatment of borderline and psychotic children', *J. Child Psychother.* 11: 87.

—— (1988) 'Beyond the unpleasure principle: some preconditions for thinking through play', *J. Child Psychother.* 14: 1–13.

Aulagnier, P. (1985) 'Il ritiro nella allucinazione: un equivalente del ritiro autistico?', *Quaderni Psicoterap. Infant.* 14: 178–194.

Balconi, M. and Del Carlo Giannini, G. (1987) *Il disegno e la psicoanalisi infantile*, Milan: Raffaello Cortina Editore.

Barale, F. (1990) 'Riflessioni a paritre dal Mosè (Trauma e storia dall'ultimo Freud a noi)', *Riv. Psicoanal.* 36: 897–919.

Barale, F. and Ferro, A. (1987) 'Sofferenza mentale dell'analista e sogni di controtransfert', *Riv. Psicoanal.* 33: 219–233.

—— (1992) 'Negative therapeutic reactions and microfractures in analytic communication', in L. Nissim Momigliano and A. Robutti (eds) *Shared Experience: The Psychoanalytic Dialogue*, London: Karnak House.

Baranger, M. and Baranger, W. (1969a) 'La situacion analitica como campo dinamico', in W. Baranger and M. Baranger *Problemas del campo psicoanalitico*, Buenos Aires: Kargieman.

—— (1969b) 'El insight en la situacion analitica', in W. Baranger and M. Baranger *Problemas del campo psicoanalitico*, Buenos Aires: Kargieman.

—— (1969c) *Problemas del campo psicoanalitico*, Buenos Aires: Kargieman.

Baranger, M., Baranger, W. and Mom, J. (1983) 'Process and non-process in analytic work', *Int. J. Psycho-Anal.* 83 (64): 1–15.

Barthes, R. (1966) 'L'analyse structurale du récit', *Communications* 8: 12–24.

Baruzzi, A. (1989) 'Presentazione', in D Meltzer, *Vita onirica*, Rome: Borla.

Bertolini, M., Geitlinger, G. and Guareschi Cazzullo, A. (1978) *Normalità, salute e malattia del bambino*, Milan: Ed. Tempo Medico.

Bettelheim, B. (1975) *The Uses of Enchantment. The Meaning and Importance of Fairy Tales*, New York: Alfred A. Knopf.

Bezoari, M. and Ferro, A. (1989) 'Listening, interpretations and transformative functions in the analytical dialogue', *Riv. Psicoanal.* 35: 1015–1051.

—— (1990) 'Elementos de un modelo del campo analitico: los agregados funcionales', *Revista de Psychoanalysis* 5(6): 847–861.

—— (1991a) 'I personaggi della seduta come aggregati funzionali del campo analitico', report to the SPI Congress, Bologna.

—— (1991b) 'From a play between parts to transformations in the couple: psychoanalysis in a bipersonal field', in L. Nissim Momigliano and A. Robutti (eds) *Shared Experience: The Psychoanalytic Dialogue*, London: Karnak House.

—— (1991c) 'L'oscillazione significati-affetti', *Riv. Psicoan.* 38(2): 380–403.

—— (1992) 'Elementos de un modelo del campo analitico: los agregados funcionales', *Revista de Psicoanalisis* 5(6): 847–861.

—— (1994) 'Listening, interpreting and psychic change in the analytic dialogue', *International Forum of Psychoanalysis* 3: 35–41.

—— (1996) 'Mots, images, affects. L'aventure du sens dans la recontre analytique', *Revue Canadienne de Psychanalyse* 4(1): 49–73.

—— (1998) 'The dream within a field theory: functional aggregates and narrations', *Journal of Melanie Klein and Object Relations* (in press).

Bick, E. (1964) 'Notes on infant observation in psycho-analytic training', *Int. J. Psycho-Anal.* 45: 558–566.

—— (1968) 'The experience of the skin in early object relation', *Int. J. Psycho-Anal.* 49: 484–486.

Bion, W.R. (1962) *Learning from Experience*, London: Heinemann.

—— (1963) *Elements of Psychoanalysis*, London: Heinemann.

—— (1965) *Transformations*, London: Heinemann.

—— (1967a) 'Hallucination', in W.R. Bion, *Second Thoughts (Select Papers of Psychoanalysis)*, London: Heinemann.

—— (1967b) 'Attacks on linkings', in W.R. Bion *Second Thoughts (Select Papers of Psychoanalysis)*, London: Heinemann.

—— (1967c) 'A theory of thinking' in W.R. Bion, *Second Thoughts (Select Papers of Psychoanalysis)*, London: Heinemann.

—— (1967d) *Second Thoughts (Select Papers of Psychoanalysis)*, London: Heinemann.

—— (1978) *Four Discussions with W.R. Bion*, Perth: Clunie Press.

—— (1980) *Bion in New York and Sao Paulo*, Perth: Clunie Press.

—— (1983) *Bion in Rome*, The Estate of W.R. Bion.

—— (1987) *Clinical Seminars and Four Papers*, The Estate of W.R. Bion.

Bion Talamo, P. (1987) 'Perché non possiamo dirci bioniani, *Gruppo e funzione analitica* 3: 279.

Bléandonu, G. (1985) *L'école de Melanie Klein*, Paris: Editions du Centurion.

Bleger, J. (1966) *Psicohigiene y psicologia institucional*, Buenos Aires: Paidos.

Bonamino, V., Di Renzo, M. and Giannotti, A. (1992) 'Le fantasie inconsce dei genitori come fattori ego-alieni nelle identificazioni del bambino', report to the Meeting of Infantile Psychoanalysis 'Identificazione e Identità nell'analisi del bambino', Rome, 8–9 February.

Bordi, S. (1980) 'Relazione analitica e sviluppo cognitivo', *Riv. Psicoanal.* 26: 161–181.

—— (1990) 'Modelli a confronto in psicoanalisi', *Prospettive psicoanalitiche nel lavoro istituzionale* 8: 71–87.

Borgogno, F. (1981) 'Osservazione: disturbo, preoccupazione, responsabilità, *Quaderni Psicoterap. Infant.* 4: 42–53.

Bott Spillius, E. (1983) 'Some developments from the work of Melanie Klein', *Int. J. Psycho-Anal.* 64: 321.

—— (ed.) (1988) *Melanie Klein Today*, 2 vols, London: Routledge.

Bremond, C. (1973) *Logique du récit*, Paris: Editions du Seuil.

Brenman, E. (1977) 'The narcissism of the analyst: its effects in clinical practise', *Psychoanalysis in Europe* 13: 20–27.

Brenman Pick, I. (1985) 'Working-through in the counter-transference', *Int. J. Psycho-Anal.* 66: 157–166.

Brutti, C. (1975) 'L'osservazione di bambino come fondamento della formazione psicologica degli operatori', in C. Brutti, *Il bambino non visto*, Rome: Editori Riuniti.

Brutti, C., Ercolani, R. and Parlani, R. (1981) 'Note sull'osservazione in un contesto istituzionale', *Quaderni Psicoterap. Infant.* 4: 113–122.

Carloni, G. (1982) 'Sofferenza psichica e vocazione terapeutica', in G. Di Chiara (ed.) *Itinerari della psicoanalisi*, Turin: Loescher.

—— (1984) 'Tatto, contatto e tattica', *Riv. Psicoanal.* 30: 191–200.

Chianese, D. (1988) 'La costruzione di una teoria. Einstein–Freud: un confronto tra modelli', *Riv. Psicoanal.* 34(3): 475.

Corrao, F. (1981) 'Introduzione', in F. Corrao, *Il cambiamento catastrofico*, Turin: Loescher.

—— (1986) 'Il concetto di campo come modello teorico', *Gruppo e funzione analitica* 7: 9–21.

—— (1988) 'Morfologia e trasformazioni nei modelli analitici', *Riv. Psicoanal.* 35: 513–543.

Corti, A. (1981) 'Da Melanie Klein a Wilfred Bion', *Riv. Psicoanal.* 27: 399–414.

Costa, A. (1979) 'L'insieme dei pazienti come oggetto interno. Il paziente come oggetto nel gruppo di lavoro', *Riv. Psicoanal.* 25: 117–126.

De Bianchedi, E.T. (1991) 'Psychic change: the "becoming" of an inquiry', *Int. J. Psycho-Anal.* 72: 6–15.

De Martis, D. (1983) 'Sui problemi della dipendenza', *Riv. Psicoanal.* 29: 296–308.

De Masi, F. (1984) 'On transference psychosis: clinical perspective in work with borderline patients', in L. Nissim Momigliano and A. Robutti (eds) *Shared Experience. The Psychoanalytic Dialogue*, London: Karnak House.

De Simone Gaburri, G. and Fornari, B. (1988) 'Melanie Klein e la scuola inglese', in A.A. Semi (ed.) *Trattato di Psicoanalisi*, vol. 1 Milan: Raffaello Cortina Editore.

De Simone Gaburri, G., Di Chiara, G. and Gaburri, E. (1981) 'Dialogo sui gruppi', *Gruppo e funzione analitica* 2: 3–12.

Di Cagno, L., Lazzarini, A., Rissone, A. and Randaccio, A. (1981) *Il neonato e il suo mondo relazionale*, Rome: Borla.

Di Chiara, G. (1982) 'L'assetto mentale dello psicoanalista quale invariante tra terapia e conoscenza', report to the VI Congress SPI, Rome.

—— (1983) 'The tale of the green hand. On projective identification', in L. Nissim Momigliano and A. Robutti (eds) *Shared Experience. The Psychoanalytic Dialogue*, London: Karnak House.

—— (1985) 'Una prospettiva psicoanalitica del dopo Freud. Un posto per l'altro', *Riv. Psicoanal.* 31: 451–462.

—— (1990) 'La stupita meraviglia, l'autismo e la competenza difensiva', *Riv. Psicoanal.* 36: 441–457.

—— (1991) 'Tradizione e sviluppi nella teoria e nella clinica psicoanalitica. Alcune considerazioni sul processo analitico'. Loveno di Menaggio, report to the I Italian–German Interview, 8 June.

—— (1992) 'Meeting, telling and parting. Three basic factors in the psychoanalytical experience', in L. Nissim Momigliano and A. Robutti (eds) *Shared Experience. The Psychoanalytic Dialogue*, London: Karnak House.

Di Chiara, G., Bogani, A., Bravi, G., Robutti, A., Viola, M. and Zanette, M. (1985) 'Preconcezione edipica e funzione psicoanalitica della mente', *Riv. Psicoanal.* 3: 237.

Di Chiara, G. and Flegenheimer, F. (1985) 'Identificazione proiettiva', *Riv. Psicoanal.* 31: 233–243.

Diderot, D. (1962/1771) 'Jacques le fataliste', in *Oeuvres romanesque*, Paris: Garnier

Dolto, F. (1948) 'Rapport sur l'interpretation psychanalytique des dessins au cours des traitements psychothérapiques', *Psyche* 17: 324–346.

Eco, U. (1981) *The Role of the Reader*, Bloomington: Indiana University Press and London: Hutchinson.

—— (1989) *The Open Work*, Cambridge: Harvard University Press.

—— (1990) *The Limits of Interpretation*, Bloomington: Indiana University Press.

Fachinelli, E. (1983) *Claustrofilia*, Milan: Adelphi.

Ferrara Mori, G., Ciampini Gazzarrini, E., Manna, A., Mazzetti, D., Root Fortini, L. and Russo, S. (1981) 'L'osservazione dell'interazione madre–bambino nel primo anno di vita', *Quaderni Psicoterap. Infant.* 4: 179–201.

Ferro, A. (1985a) 'Capacità di rêverie, contenimento e rapporto oggettuale nella mente dell'analista di bambini', *Psichiatria dell'infanzia e dell'adolescenza* 52: 505–514.

—— (1985b) 'L'osservazione del gioco infantile', *Psichiatria dell'infanzia e dell'adolescenza* 52: 295–300.

—— (1985c) 'Psicoanalisi e favole', *Riv. Psicoanal.* 31: 216–230.

—— (1985d) 'Riflessioni su alcune oscillazioni nella relazione analitica attraverso una analisi infantile', *Psichiatria dell'infanzia e dell'adolescenza* 52: 163–171.

—— (1986) 'Da Robot a Pinocchio: lento cammino di una trasformazione', *Psichiatria dell'infanzia e dell'adolescenza* 53: 171–185.

—— (1987a) 'Il mondo alla rovescia. L'inversione di flusso delle identificazioni proiettive', *Riv. Psicoanal.* 33: 59–77.

—— (1987b) 'L'analisi di un bambino come luogo per evidenziare le identificazioni proiettive del terapeuta', *Psichiatria dell'infanzia e dell'adolescenza* 54: 3–7.

—— (1988) 'Dall'allucinazione al sogno: dall'evacuazione alla tollerabilità del dolore', *Pschiatria dell'infanzia e dell'adolescenza* 55: 733–744.

—— (1991) 'From Raging Bull to Theseus: the long path of a transformation', *Int. J. Psycho-Anal.* 72: 417–425.

—— (1993a) 'Disegno, identificazione proiettiva e processi trasformativi', *Riv. Psicoanal.* 39(4): 667–680.

—— (1993b) 'From hallucination to dream: from evacuation to the tolerability of pain in the analysis of a preadolescent', *Psychoanalytic Review* 80(3): 389–404.

—— (1993c) 'The impasse within a theory of the analytic field: possible vertices of observation', *Int. J. Psycho-Anal.* 74(5): 971–929.

—— (1994) 'Two authors in search of characters: the relationship, the field, the story', *Australian Journal of Psychoterapy* 13, 1–1.

—— (1996) 'Carla's panic attacks: insight and transformations: what comes out of the cracks: monster or nascent thoughts?', *Int. J. Psycho-Anal.* 77: 997–1011.

—— (1997) 'L'unicit de l'analyse entre analogres et différences dans l'analyse d'enfants et d'adolescents', *Psychanalyse en Europe Bulletin FEP* 50: 49–60.

—— (1998a) 'The unity of the analysis underlying the similarities and differences in the analysis of children and adolescents', Bulletin 50, European Psychoanalytical Federation.

—— (1998b) '"Characters" and their precursors in depression: experiences and transformation in the course of therapy', *International Journal of Melanie Klein and Object Relations* (in press).

Ferro, A., Pasquali, G., Tognoli, L. and Viola, M. (1986a) 'L'uso del simbolismo nel setting e il processo di simbolizzazione del pensiero psicoanalitico', *Riv. Psicoanal.* 32: 539–553.

—— (1986b) 'Note sul processo di simbolizzazione nel pensiero psicoanalitico', *Riv. Psicoanal.* 32: 521–538.

Flegenheimer, F.A. (1983) 'Divergenze e punti comuni tra psicoanalisi infantile e psicoanalisi degli adulti: alcune riflessioni', *Riv. Psicoanal.* 29: 196–205.

Fornari, F. (1963) *La vita affettiva originaria del bambino*, Milan: Feltrinelli.

—— (1975) Genialità e cultura, Milan: Feltrinelli.

Freud, A. (1936) *The Ego and the Mechanism of Defence*, London: Hogarth Press.

—— (1946) *The Psycho-Analytical Treatment of Children (1926–1945)*, London: Imago.

Freud, S. (1899) 'Die Traumdeutung', *Gesammelte Werke 2–3*, Vienna.

—— (1906) *Der Wann und die Traume in Wilhelm Jensens 'Gradiva'*, G.W. 7.

—— (1908) *Analyse der Phobie eines Fünfjährigen Knaben*, G.W. 7.

—— (1909) *Bemerkungen über einen Fall von Zwangsneurose*, G.W. 7.

—— (1920) *Jenseits des Lustprinzips*, G.W. 13.

—— (1924) *Notiz über den 'Wunderblock'*, G.W. 14.

—— (1932) *Neue Folge der Vorlesungen zur Einführung in die Psychoanalyse*, G.W. 15.

Gaburri, E. (1982) 'Una ipotesi di relazione tra trasgressione e pensiero', *Riv. Psicoanal.* 4: 511.

—— (1987) 'Dal gemello immaginario al compagno segreto', *Riv. Psicoanal.* 32, 4: 509–620.

—— (1992) Personal communication.

Gaburri, E. and Ferro, A. (1988) 'Gli sviluppi kleiniani e Bion', in A.A. Semi (ed.) *Trattato di psicoanalisi*, vol. 1, Milan: Raffaello Cortina Editore.

Gaddini, E. (1976) 'Discussion of the role of family life in child development', *Int. J. Psycho-Anal.* 57: 397–409.

—— (1989) *Scritti 1953–1985*, Milan: Raffaello Cortina Editore.

Gagliardi Guidi, R. (1992) 'Premature termination of analysis', in L. Nissim Momigliano and A. Robutti (eds) *Shared Experience. The Psychoanalytic Dialogue*. London: Karnak House.

Gear, H.C., Grinberg, L. and Liendo, E.C. (1976) *Group Dynamics According to a Semiotic*

Model Based on Projective and Counterprojective Identification, New York: Group Therapy Stratton Intercontinental.

Generali Clements, L. (1971) 'L'osservazione del neonato come metodo di studio in psichiatria infantile', *Riv. Psicoanal.* 1: 173.

—— (1983) 'I sogni a occhi aperti di Kathrina: identificazione proiettiva come attacco e come comunicazione', *Riv. Psicoanal.* 29: 213–226.

Generali Clements, L. and Ferrara Mori, G. (1980) 'Correlazioni tra la relazione analitica e la relazione madre–bambino', report to the VI Congress SPI, Taormina.

Giannotti, A. and De Astis, G. (1989) *Il disegnale. Psicopatologia degli stati precoci dello sviluppo*, Rome: Borla.

Green, A. (1973) *Le discours vivant/La conception psychanalytique de l'Affect*, Paris: Presses Universitaires de France.

Greenson, R.R. (1967) *The Technique and Practise of Psychoanalysis*, London: Hogarth Press.

Greimas, A. (1966) *Sémantique Structurale*, Paris: Larousse.

—— (1983) *Du Sens*, Paris: Editions du Seuil.

Grinberg, L., Sor, D. and Tabak de Bianchedi, R. (1975) *Introduction to the Work of Bion*, Perth: Clunie Press.

Hamon, P. (1972) 'Pour un statut semiologique du personnage', *Littérature*, 6.

Harris, M. (1987) *A Baby Observation: The Absent Object. Collected papers of Martha Harris and Esther Bick*, Perth: Clunie Press.

Hautmann, G. (1965) 'Un esempio di controidentificazione proiettiva', *Riv. Psicoanal.* 11: 247–266.

—— (1977) 'Pensiero onirico e realtà psichica', *Riv. Psicoanal.* 23: 63-127.

Hug-Hellmuth, H. (1921) 'Zur Technik der Kinder-Analyse', *Int. Zeit. für Psychoanalyse* 7: 2.

Isaacs, S. (1948) 'The nature and function of phantasy', in J. Riviere (ed.) *Developments in Psychoanalysis*, London: Hogarth Press.

Joseph, B. (1984) 'Projective identification: clinical aspects', in J. Sandeer (ed.) *Projection, Identification, Projective Identifications*, Madison CT: International Universities Press.

—— (1985) 'Transference: the total situation', *Int. J. Psychoanal.* 66: 447–454.

—— (1989) *Psychic Equilibrium and Psychic Change*, London: Routledge.

Kafka, F. (1961) *Metamorphosis*, trans. W. and E. Muir, London: Penguin.

Klauber, G. (1979) *Difficulties in the Analytic Encounters*, New York and London: Jason Arotson.

Klein, M. (1926a) 'Infant analysis', *International Journal of Psycho-Analysis* 7: 371–373.

—— (1926b) 'The psychological principles of infant analysis', *Int. J. Psycho-Anal.* 8: 25–37.

—— (1927a) 'Criminal tendencies in normal children', *British Journal of Medical Psychology* 7: 177–192.

—— (1927b) 'Symposium on child analysis', *Int. J. Psycho-Anal.* 8: 339–370.

—— (1928) 'Early stages of the Oedipus conflict', *Int. J. Psycho-Anal.* 9: 167–180.

—— (1929) 'Personification in the play of children, *Int. J. Psycho-Anal.* 10: 193–204.

—— (1930) 'The importance of symbol-formation in the development of the ego', *Int. J. Psycho-Anal.* 11: 24–39.

—— (1932) *The Psychoanalysis of Children*, London: Hogarth Press.

—— (1934) 'On criminality', *British Journal of Medical Psychology* 14: 312–315.

—— (1945) 'The Oedipus complex in the light of early anxieties', *Int. J. Psycho-Anal.* 26: 11–33.

—— (1946) 'Notes on some schizoid mechanisms', *Int. J. Psycho-Anal.* 27: 99–110.

—— (1952a) 'The origins of transference', *Int. J. Psycho-Anal.* 33: 433–438.

—— (1952b) 'On observing the behaviour of young infants', in M. Klein, P. Heimann, S. Isaacs and J. Riviere *Developments in Psycho-Analysis*, London: Hogarth Press.

—— (1957) *Envy and gratitude*, in *Writings*, vol. 3, Envy and gratitude and other works (1975), London: Hogarth Press and Institute of Psycho-Analysis.

—— (1959) *Our Adult World and Other Essays*, London: Heinemann.

—— (1961) *Narrative of a Child Analysis. The Conduct of the Psycho-Analysis of Children as Seen in the Treatment of a Ten Year Old Boy*, London: Hogarth Press.

Klein, S. (1980) 'Autistic phenomena in neurotic patients', *Int. J. Psycho-Anal.* 61: 395.

Klein, M., Heimann, P. and Money-Kyrle, R.E. (1955) *New Directions in Psychoanalysis: The Significance of Infant Conflict in the Pattern of Adult Behaviour*, London: Tavistock.

Langs, R. (1975) 'The patient's unconscious perception of the therapist's errors', in P.L. Giovacchini (ed.) *Tactics and Techniques in Psychoanalytic Therapy, Vol. 2: Countertransference*, New York: Jason Aronson.

—— (1978) 'Interventions in the bipersonal field', in R. Langs, *Techniques in Transition*, New York: Jason Aronson.

—— (1984) 'The contributions of the adaptional interactional approach to classical psychoanalysis', *Analytic Psychotherapy and Psychopathology* 1: 21–47.

Lebovici, S. and McDougall, J. (1960) *Un cas de psychose infantile (étude psychanalytique)*, Paris: Presses Universitaires de France.

Leonardi, P. (1987) 'Pensiero, specificità degli oggetti e onniscenza', *Riv. Psicoanal.* 33: 321–330.

Lichtmann, A. (1990) 'Vigencia de las teorias kleinianas en el psicoanalisis actual', *Revista de Psicoanalisis* 47(2): 230.

Lussana, P. (1983) 'Sentirsi capito e sollevato: su Richard e il senso dell'analisi kleiniana, ricordando una visita a M. Klein', *Riv. Psicoanal.* 29: 132–142.

—— (1989) 'La psicoanalisi infantile su base kleiniana', in A.A. Semi (ed.) *Trattato di psicoanalisi*, vol. 2, Milan: Raffaello Cortina Editore.

—— (1991) 'Dall'interpretazione kleiniana all'interpretazione bioniana, attraverso l'osservazione dell'infantile', report to the AIPPL, Rome, 2 June.

—— (1992a) 'Evoluzione delle qualità e funzioni del contenitore-seno nell'analisi di un tredicenne e nella Madonna con Bambino del Caravaggio', in P. Lussana, *L'adolescente, lo psicoanalista, l'artista, una visione binoculare della adolescenza*, Rome: Borla.

—— (1992b) *L'adolescente, lo psicoanalista, l'artista, una visione binoculare dell'adolescenza*, Rome: Borla.

Magagna, J. (1987) 'Three years of infant observation with Mrs. Bick', *J. Child Psychother.* 13: 1.

Maldonado, J.L. (1984) 'Analyst involvement in the psychoanalytical impasse', *Int. J. Psycho-Anal.* 65: 263–271.

—— (1987) 'Narcissism and unconscious communication', *Int. J. Psycho-Anal.* 68: 379–387.

Mancia, M. (1984) 'Memoria, simbolizzazione e funzioni del sogno', report to the VI Congress SPI, Taormina.

—— (1987) *Il sogno come religione della mente*, Rome-Bari: Laterza.

Manfredi Turillazzi, S. (1978) 'Interpretazione dell'agire e interpretazione come agire', *Riv. Psicoanal.* 24: 223–240.

—— (1985) 'L'unicorno. Saggio sulla fantasia e l'oggetto nel concetto di identificazione proiettiva', *Riv. Psicoanal.* 31: 462–477.

Manfredi Turillazzi, S. and Ferro, A. (1990) 'Introduzione', in S. Manfredi Tutillazzi and A. Ferro, *La situazione psicoanalitica come campo bipersonale*, Milan: Raffello Cortina Editore.

Meltzer, D. (1964) *Eight Lectures on Child Analysis*, unpublished paper.

—— (1965) 'The relation of anal masturbation to projective identification', *Int. J. Psycho-Anal.* 47: 335–342.

—— (1967) *The Psychoanalytic Process*, London: Heinemann.

—— (1973) *Sexual States of Mind*, Perth: Clunie Press.

—— (1974) 'Adhesive identification', *Contemporary Psycho-Analysis* 11: 289–310.

—— (1976) 'Routine and inspired interpretations', *Contemporary Psycho-Analysis* 14: 210–225.

—— (1978a) *The Kleinian Development*, London: Donald Meltzer.

—— (1978b) 'A note on Bion's concept "reversal of alpha-function"', in D. Meltzer, *The Kleinian Development*, London: Donald Meltzer, 119–129.

—— (1979) 'Posizione schizoparanoide e posizione depressiva', *Quaderni Psicoterap. Infant.* 1: 125–141.

—— (1981a) 'Del simbolo', *Quaderni Psicoterap. Infant.*, 5.

—— (1981b) 'The Kleinian explosion of Freud's metapsychology', *Int. J. Psycho-Anal.* 62: 177–185.

—— (1982a) 'Una indagine sulle bugie: loro genesi e relazione con l'allucinazione', *Quaderni Psicoterap. Infant.* 13: 187–191.

—— (1982b) 'Verità della mente e bugia nella vita del sogno', *Quaderni Psicoterap. Infant.* 13: 139–160.

—— (1982c) 'Interventi in allucinazione e bugia', *Quaderni Psicoterap. Infant.* 13: 161–175.

—— (1984) *Dream Life*, Perth: Clunie Press.

—— (1986a) 'Riflessione sui mutamenti nel mio metodo psicoanalitico', *Psicoterapia e scienze umane* 20: 260–269.

—— (1986b) *Studies in Extended Metapsychology*, Perth: Clunie Press.

Meltzer, D. and Harris, M. (1983) *Child, Family and Community: A Psychoanalytical Model of Learning Process*, Paris: OECD.

Meotti, A. (1984) 'Di alcuni orientamenti della psicoanalisi italiana. Note e considerazioni su una recente raccolta di studi psicoanalitici', *Riv. Psicoanal.* 30: 109–121.

—— (1990) Personal communication.

Meotti, A. and Meotti, F. (1983) 'Su alcuni aspetti dei processi riparativi', *Riv. Psicoanal.* 28: 227–242.

Miller, A. (1979) *Das Drama des begabten Kinders*, Frankfurt: Suhrkamp Verlag.

—— (1981) *Du sollst nicht merken: Variationen über das Paradies-Thema*, Frankfurt: Suhrkamp Verlag.

Milner, M. (1969) *The Hands of the Living God. An Account of a Psycho-Analytic Treatment*, London: Hogarth Press.

Molinari Negrini, S. (1985) 'Funzione di testimonianza e interpretazioni di transfert', *Riv. Psicoanal.* 30(3): 357–371.

Molinari Negrini, S. (1991) Personal communication.

Money-Kyrle, R. (1956) 'Normal counter-transference and some of its deviations', *Int. J. Psycho-Anal.* 37: 360–366.

―― (1978) 'Success and failure in mental maturations', in R. Money-Kyrle, *The Collected Papers of Roger Money-Kyrle*, Perth: Clunie Press, 397–406.

Morgenstern, S. (1937) *Psychanalyse infantile*, Paris: Denoel.

Morra, M. (1983) 'Freud e Klein: applicazioni nella clinica', *Riv. Psicoanal.* 29: 206–212.

Muratori, A.M. and Cargnelutti, E. (1988) 'Trasformazioni in psicoanalisi', *Riv. Psicoanal.* 34(3): 454–473.

Musatti, C. (1949) *Trattato di psicoanalisi*, Turin: Boringhieri.

Negri, R. (1987) 'L'osservazione del neonato: metodologia di studio dei processi mentali', *Quaderni Psicoterap. Infant.* 18: 100–116.

―― (1991) 'L'osservazione del neonato gravemente pretermine', Atti del I Colloque europeéen 'L'observation du nourisson et ses applications', Brussels, 26 October.

Neri, C., Correale, A. and Fadda, P. (1987) *Letture bioniane*, Rome: Borla.

Neri, C., Pallier, L., Petacchi, G., Soavi, G.C. and Tagliacozzo, R. (1989) 'Dal rifiuto all'accettazione nelle analisi degli adulti (teoria e tecnica)', *Riv. Psicoanal.* 35: 781–785.

Nissim Momigliano, L. (1981) 'La memoria e il desiderio', *Riv. Psicoanal.* 27(4): 533–544.

―― (1984) 'Two people talking in a room: an investigation on the analytic dialogue', in L. Nissim Momigliano and A. Robutti (eds) *Shared Experience. The Psychoanalytic Dialogue*, London: Karnak House.

―― (1987) 'A spell in Vienna: but was Freud a Freudian?, *Int. Rev. Psycho-Anal.* 14(3): 373–389.

Nissim Momigliano, L. and Robutti, A. (eds) (1991) *Shared Experience. The Psychoanalytic Dialogue*. London: Karnak House.

Ogden, T.H. (1979) 'On projective identification', *Int. J. Psycho-Anal.* 60: 357–373.

―― (1982) Projective Identification and Psychotherapeutic Technique, New York: Jason Aronson.

Petrella, F. (1988) 'Il modello freudiano', in A.A. Semi (ed.) *Trattato di psicoanalisi*, vol. 1, Milan: Raffaello Cortina Editore.

Pichon-Riviere, E. (1971) *El proceso grupal*, Buenos Aires: Nueva Vision.

Pierloot, R.A. (1987) 'The analysand as a character in search of an author', *Int. Rev. Psycho-Anal.* 14: 221.

Piontelli, A. (1986) *Backwards in Time: A Study in Infant Observation by the Method of Esther Bick*, London: Karnak House.

Propp, V. (1969) *Morphology of the Folk Tales*, Houston: University of Texas.

Rambert, M. (1938) 'Une nouvelle technique en psychanalyse infantile: le jeu des guignols', *Revue Française de Psychanalyse* 10: 581–595.

Resnik, S. (1982) *Il teatro del sogno*, Turin: Boringhieri.

Riolo, F. (1983) 'Sogno e teoria della conoscenza in psicoanalisi', *Riv. Psicoanal.* 29: 279–295.

Riviere, J. (ed.) (1952) *Developments in Psychoanalysis*, London: Hogarth Press.

Robutti, A. (1991) 'Introduction', in L. Nissim Momigliano and A. Robutti (eds) *Shared Experience. The Psychoanalytic Dialogue*, London: Karnak House.

Rosenfeld, H. (1987) *Impasse and Interpretation*, London: Tavistock.

Rothstein, A. (ed.) (1985) *Models of the Mind. Their Relationship to Clinical Work*, Madison CT: International Universities Press.

Saraval, A. (1985) 'L'analista può essere neutrale?', *Riv. Psicoanal.* 31: 343–356.

Schafer, R. (ed.) (1997) *The Contemporary Kleinians of London*, Madison CT: International Universities Press.

Schlesinger, C. (1989) 'Del metroide', *Riv. Psicoanal.* 35: 141–169.

Segal, H. (1957) 'Notes on symbol formation', *Int. J. Psycho-Anal.* 38: 391–397.

—— (1978) 'On symbolism', *Int. J. Psycho-Anal.* 59: 315.

—— (1979) *M. Klein*, London: Fontana.

—— (1983) 'Some clinical implication of Melanie Klein's work', *Int. J. Psycho-Anal.* 64: 269.

—— (1985) 'The Kleinian–Bion Model', in A. Rothstein (ed.) *Models of the Mind*, Madison CT: International Universities Press.

Semi, A.A. (ed.) (1988–9) *Trattato di psicoanalisi*, 2 vols, Milan: Raffaello Cortina Editore.

Sharpe, E. (1937) *Dream Analysis*, London: Hogarth Press.

Siniavsky, M. (1979) 'Acerca de la identitad del analista de niños su ruptura y desercion', *Psicoanalisis* 2: 2–14.

Sklovskij, V. (1925) *O teorii prozy*, Moscow.

Speziale Bagliacca, R. (1982) *Sulle spalle di Freud*, Rome: Astrolabio.

—— (1991) 'The capacity to contain: notes on its function in psychic change', *Int. J. Psycho-Anal.* 72: 27.

—— (ed.) (1988) *Melanie Klein Today*, 2 vols, London: Routledge.

Sponitz, H. (1969) *Modern Psychoanalysis of the Schizophrenic Patient*, New York: Grune and Stratton.

Stern, D.N. (1977) *The First Relationship: Infant and Mother*, Cambridge MA: Harvard University Press.

—— (1985) *The Interpersonal World of the Infant*, New York: Basic Books.

Tagliacozzo, R. (1982) 'La pensabilità: una meta della psicoanalisi', in G. Di Chiara (ed.) *Itinerari della psicoanalisi*, Turin: Loescher.

—— (1990) 'Cercare di pensare con Freud', *Riv. Psicoanal.* 36: 804–829.

Taylor, D. (1983) 'Some observations on hallucinations', *Int. J. Psycho-Anal.* 64: 3.

Todorov, T. (1965) *Théorie de la littérature. Textes des formalistes russes*, Paris: Seuil.

—— (1971) *Poétique de la prose*, Paris: Seuil.

—— (1975) 'La lecture comme construction', *Poetique*, 24: 417–425.

Tomasevskij, B. (1928) *Teorija literatury. Poetikan*, Leningrad.

Torras de Bea, E. and Rallo Romero, J. (1986) 'Past and present interpretation', *Int. Rev. Psycho-Anal.* 13: 309.

Tustin, F. (1986) *Autistic Barriers in Neurotic Patients*, London: Karnak House.

Tynjanon, J. (1965) 'Problema stickotvornogo jazyka' in T. Todorov *Théorie de la littérature*, Paris: Sevil.

Vallino Macciò, D. (1981) 'Ansia di separazione rilevata nell'osservazione del neonato e nella psicoanalisi di adolescenti e adulti', *Giorn. Neuropsich. Età Evol.* 1(2): 173–184.

—— (1984) 'Sulla terminabilità di una analisi infantile che raggiunge l'adolescenza. Contributo clinico', *Riv. Psicoanal.* 30(34): 387–397.

—— (1990) 'Sulla consultazione: atmosfere emotive, sofferenza e sollievo del bambino', *Analysis* 1: 325–335.

—— (1991) 'Il gioco delle parti nella reverie dell'analista', report to the IX Congresso SPI, Saint Vincent.

—— (1992) 'Surviving, existing, living. Notes on the analyst's anxiety', in L. Nissim

Momigliano and A. Robutti (eds) *Shared Experience. The Psychoanalytic Dialogue*, London: Karnak House.

Vallino Macciò, D., Bertone, P., Crivelli, E., Pozzi, A. and Nacinovich, R. (1990) 'Risonanze affettive e professionalità dell'educatore', in A. Costantino, and M. Noziglia (eds) *Osservazione del bambino e formazione degli educatori*, Milano: Unicopli.

Vattimo, G. (1983) 'Dialettica, differenza, pensiero debole', in G.Vattimo and P.A. Rovatti (eds) *Il pensiero debole*, Milano: Feltrinelli.

Vergine, A. (1991) 'Riflessioni generali sul tema del Congresso', report to the ninth national IX Congress SPI 'Gli affetti', Saint Vincent, Rome: Borla.

Waksman, J. (1985) 'La controtransferencia de l'analista de niños', Psicoanalisis 7: 3.

Wallerstein, R. (1988) 'One psychoanalysis or many?', *Int. J. Psycho-Anal.* 69: 5–21.

Widlocher, D. (1965) *L'interpretation des dessins d'enfants*, Brussels: Charles Dessart.

Widlocher, D. and Engelhart, D. (1975) 'Dessins et psychopathologie de l'enfant', *La psychiatrie de l'enfant*, 18(2): 315–398.

Winnicott, D.W. (1949) 'Hate in the countertransference', *Int. J. Psycho-Anal*, 30: 69–74.

—— (1965) *The Maturational Processes and Facilitating Environment*, London: Hogarth Press.

—— (1971a) *Therapeutic Consultations in Child Psychiatry*, London: Hogarth Press.

—— (1971b) *Playing and Reality*, London: Tavistock.

Index